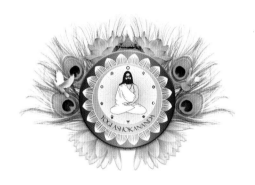

THE POWER OF
RELAXATION

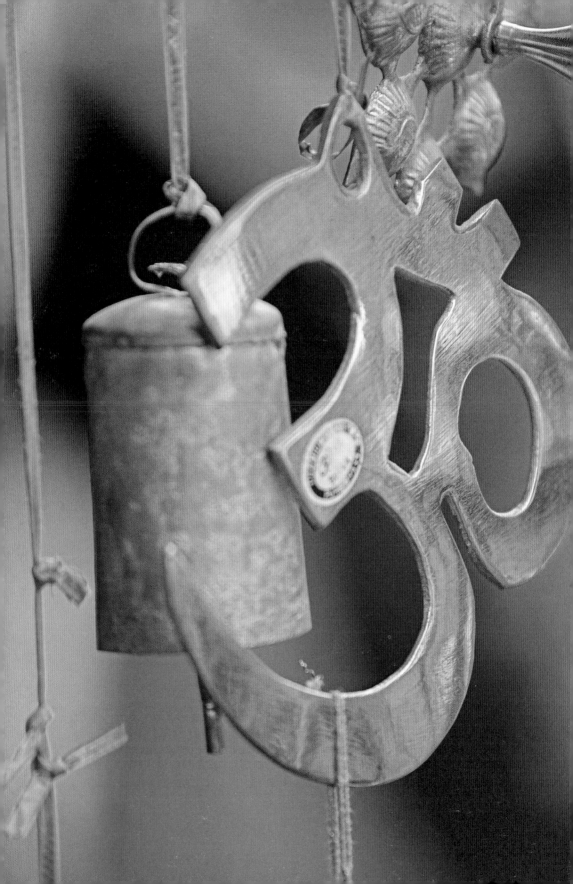

THE POWER OF RELAXATION

Align your body, your mind
and your life through meditation

YOGI ASHOKANANDA

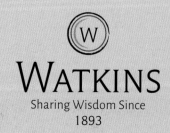

WATKINS

Sharing Wisdom Since
1893

The Power of Relaxation
Yogi Ashokananda

First published in the UK and USA in 2015 by
Watkins Media Limited
19 Cecil Court
London, WC2N 4HE

enquiries@watkinspublishing.co.uk

Managing Editor: Sandra Rigby
Senior Editor: Fiona Robertson
Editor: Jane McIntosh
Art Director: Georgina Hewitt
Designer: Luana Gobbo
Commissioned Photography: Christina Wilson
Picture Research: Cee Weston-Baker
Production: Uzma Taj

A CIP record for this book is available from the British Library

ISBN: 978-1-78028-714-0

10 9 8 7 6 5 4 3 2 1

Typeset in Agenda and Goudy
Colour reproduction by XY Digital
Printed in China

www.watkinspublishing.com

Contents

Introduction

Nowadays everybody wants to experience meditation through yoga, but traditionally it was the other way round – yoga (yuj) was experienced by practising meditation. I do not think of my own practice as a prescription for my life or a hobby that I can discuss at a dinner party. Instead, I integrate yoga and meditation into my life and live them along with everything else.

On my first and second visits to London I felt overwhelmed and drained because I had never before experienced a metropolis like this. I described my reaction to my teacher and he replied, 'You don't know how to meditate.' And so I made a plan ... I looked for the busiest place in London and discovered it on Oxford Street. I set myself the task of meditating there during peak shopping hours. I found a spot and stood still, trying to meditate (I didn't sit down because I didn't want to draw attention to myself). I did this until I was able to rediscover the silence within me amid all the external bustle. Once I had reached a place of inner silence and found the peace that exists within, I was oblivious to my surroundings – I couldn't hear a thing and nothing could bother me!

I have lived in the UK since 2005, teaching various techniques and practices (including those featured in this book, as well as others) in order to help people connect with themselves and find a sense of balance with everything around them. These methods provide the tools to leave behind uneasy circumstances and situations, to grow, and to live a healthier and happier life. My teaching comes from years of study, practice and experience alongside my teachers, my friends and all my students. I feel it is important to honour the traditions and stay true to the roots of these practices, which came from ancient yogis. Although I have been able to adapt these methods to suit the lives of people in the 21st century, they have not lost any of their authenticity and sacredness.

In India, my teacher, the late Gurudev Dilipji, and I taught many of these practices, with some amazing results. A number of people helped me in this

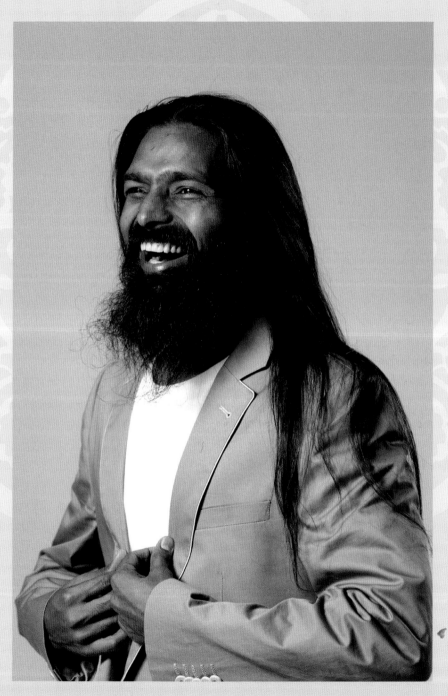

Yogi Ashokananda's practice is based on embracing the whole self, with all its desires, disappointments, confusion, pain, love and joy.

by giving me instruction and encouragement. They include: my Guruji, Swami Vishwarupananda; Dandi Swami Sri Hansananda Saraswati (god brother of Maharishi Mahesh Yogi); the late Sri Krishna Ojha; Masta Baba (the funniest, strongest character in my life); my beloved grandfather, the late Sri Lalji; and, of course, my beloved friends. I deeply appreciate the help of Mary Attwood in collecting and writing up these teachings for this book; she is a creative visionary!

The practices in this book have been highly effective in my own life, helping me through difficult personal circumstances and healing emotional wounds. Hurt feelings, disappointment, confusion and desire are common to all human beings. These emotions can leave a person scarred or in pain, to a degree that depends on the individual's own awareness. Many people experience psychological problems when trying to follow spiritual techniques and practices. These problems are partly the result of poor teaching, but also arise when someone is thrown too quickly into a deep inner state without establishing psychological stability first.

I have met people who thought they could change themselves through spiritual practice or by joining a spiritual group, but nothing shifted inside them. All they did was become 'spiritually bipolar' and increasingly frustrated at the inconsistency between the life they imagined for themselves and the life they were living in reality. New Age thinking is often responsible for this state of affairs as it deals primarily with instant results and encourages shopping around for spirituality. It tells us that we can heal ourselves, or distract ourselves from the symptoms or causes of unhappiness or dis-ease, by acquiring a new identity as a positive thinker. But true spiritual growth is not about quick fixes and replacement; it requires patience, acceptance and transformation.

When we acquire a new belief system or thought process, we are often under the impression that we have to think positively all the time. This is both unrealistic and exhausting! When I came to the West it really struck me that so many people feel guilty about having negative emotions and try to 'cleanse' themselves of these thoughts or feelings.

A path to your authentic self

The practices I share in this book allow you to relax into your authentic self without the pressure of having to be 'happy' all the time. Ironically, when this pressure is taken away, we feel more content and fulfilled. We become more aware of our own patterns of behaviour, and the split between our material personality and our spiritual self is healed.

As our world becomes increasingly frenetic, it is ever more important to find inner stillness. Even when we go on a retreat or to a peaceful place, our surroundings may be quiet but we are not necessarily quiet within. My practices are based on embracing the whole self and trying to create a sense of humanity. This happens by accepting and transforming the lower three chakras, concerned with grounding, rootedness, mental and physical constipation, anger, sexuality, self-confidence, greed and lust. Your spirit or soul is already perfect and whole – it does not require healing. All it needs is space for you to experience your highest self. You will accomplish this by clearing the physical and emotional pathways to it and ridding yourself of samskaras (the imprints in your personality of unused emotions from experiences – see page 33).

We constantly separate, classify and label everything in life – religion, politics, society and so on – and this creates conflict. The body, too, is viewed as something separate rather than as part of us. People who think that meditation happens only in the mental body are running away from their present experience. I believe meditation happens *through the body*, and that in order for our awareness to shine, we must engage our senses and the body's present state. The tangible body is a gateway into the non-tangible part of ourselves. Without it we cannot achieve total relaxation.

I grew up in a village in northern India, where people lived in a simple, natural way. Most of the villagers owned very little, but there was a strong sense of community. If someone had grown vegetables, they would always give some away. Village life was basic but there was an abundance of love and a sharing of resources. We were surrounded by nature, and the silence and stillness after sunset was profound. I used to watch animals engaging in their own activities without noticing anyone around them, and through this physical expression of centredness I sensed a larger force at play in the world.

I saw unity in the simplicity of the villagers' way of life. As time went on, people started to acquire televisions and other appliances, and the atmosphere changed. The village lost its sense of community because desirable objects became the focus of people's attention rather than the relationships between each other. We can see this happening the world over. The material things, which are there to support us in life, become the primary focus of our life.

I was first introduced to yoga as a young child by my grandfather, who practised on a sack cloth. I saw the difference that yoga and meditation could make to my life, and they have been part of it ever since. My yoga teachers taught me many techniques and practices, but one of the most valuable lessons I learned was patience.

I don't stick to a rigid routine of always practising at the same time. Just as I drink when I'm thirsty, eat when I'm hungry and sleep when I'm tired, I practise every day, but the time varies according to my schedule and how I feel. As for self-discipline, I don't suppress things – I experience them, I feel them. For me, being mindful and aware is practising self-discipline. I listen to myself – setting conditions for my practice would only mean I was exchanging one set of mental shackles for another.

When you embark on a new journey of yoga and meditation, it is easy to set yourself up to feel guilty if you miss a practice. Just be open to your own feelings and emotions – in other words, do not deny any part of yourself. The experience of finding the centre of yourself, your self-religion, is known as swadharma. From this place I feel centred to share my experiences and help others to heal on any level, whether the discomfort is physical, emotional or spiritual.

Many people have pre-determined and fixed expectations of what it is to live a spiritual life – or one that is focused on material concerns. Many spiritual people think material people are shallow, and many material people think that a spiritual person should lead a very simple existence, liberated from earthly concerns, suppressing desires – and being miserable! I once had someone from India come to visit me in England (he turned up wanting me to teach him). At the time I was living in London in someone's beautiful garden shed and I was happy. When the visitor arrived I was cleaning my floor and singing along to a recording of John Denver's song 'All This Joy'. My visitor was totally shocked to find me singing a Western song. He had expected me to be something else, but his perception had nothing to do with me or my ability or experience.

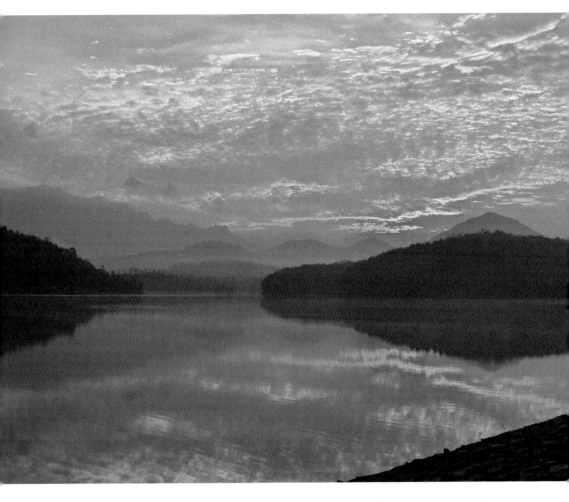

Neyyar Dam, Kerala (photograph by Yogi Ashokananda). To achieve true relaxation, we must mirror the stillness that exists in nature with a stillness within ourselves.

Finding peace at the physical level and not running away from yourself in your mind (which can often happen with still forms of meditation) is key. My practices will help you to find a long-lasting peace within yourself that allows you to be with all your emotions and feelings without the gloss of 'positive thinking'. In this way you can be your true, authentic self, connected and compassionate with yourself as well as others. Many people have found the effects of the meditation practices in this book to be profound and life-altering.

How to Use This Book

The following pages provide a brief chapter summary and explain how to approach the exercises. This book takes you through a complete process of relaxation and should therefore be read in chapter order. However, you should approach the exercises in order of difficulty (see opposite). These exercises will help you to find patience and stillness, and aid the transformation within.

In one way or another we are all searching for power or strength. It is important to know what real power is and what takes power away from you. Chapter 1 lays the foundations for understanding what true power is, what controls it and how you can rediscover your power and connect with it.

Chapter 2 is focused on the breath, as this is the fundamental element that connects you to your inner power. If your mind is not aligned to the power and creativity inside you, these will remain locked away from you. Through your breath you can gain a clear, focused and steady mind that will connect you to your inner treasure. Your breath also brings you vitality and refreshes your spirit. Your breath gives you stamina and the ability to cope in stressful and difficult situations. Whatever emotion you feel – fear, anxiety or joy – its first effect is on your breath, and this in turn affects your mind, your spirit and your power.

Chapter 3 is concerned with the power within the body. Your breath exists in the body, your mind exists in the body and your power exists in the body. As your individual power exists within your individual body, it is important to get to know your physical body in order to be able to release trapped energy and stimulate the creation of energy.

Chapter 4 introduces primordial sound. Your body is filled with microscopic hollow spaces – and these spaces contain the frequency of primordial sound. In this chapter your inner voice is revealed and your inner frequency aligned with your outer frequency so that you feel whole. By connecting your individual frequency to the universal frequency you are able to see the truth.

Chapter 5 explores the meaning of duality and looks at how opposite forces – the material and the spiritual – are inherent in our lives. This chapter stresses the need to accept your positive *and* your negative traits, and it gives you the mental strength to stay focused on your practice while also accepting your indecision and the self-questioning and self-doubts. This is duality.

Having experienced the techniques and practices of the previous chapters, by Chapter 6 you should be feeling much more centred in yourself, accepting the duality of your nature. By connecting to your inner voice, by accepting and embracing your body, by controlling your breath and by knowing that your breath controls your power, you can remain in your centre. You can access a state of total relaxation and carry this with you wherever you are and wherever you go.

All the exercises have the same ultimate aim – to bring you back to yourself – and there are different techniques or pathways to this. Exercises are rated for difficulty using a colour-coded lotus flower (see page 14), because some are much more effective once you have developed the lung capacity, physical stamina, and mental and psychological attunement necessary to do them. In addition, this gradual approach will help you to develop patience and mindfulness with the here-and-now. Ask yourself every day: 'How much time do I have?', 'What do I need to do for myself?', 'When will I feed myself?'. You should also consider which exercises you feel naturally drawn to.

Choose a time and a place for your meditation where you will not be disturbed. Switch off your mobile phone. If you do not have time for yourself, create it!

I would suggest doing the orange exercises first. Practise any of these every day (or as and when you can, but at least once a week) for a month before moving on to the next set. Progress through the yellow and green exercises. (It is OK to continue to practise any of the orange exercises alongside the harder ones.) Finally, practise the advanced, blue exercises, which to be their most effective require you to have done the groundwork with the previous exercises.

To help you in your practice, you can download a recording of Awakening the Primordial Sound (page 110), the Gayatri Mantra (page 114), Stitching Together Left and Right (pages 132–4), Rising Sap (pages 135–7) and the Science of Relaxation™ meditation (pages 148–51), all from www.yogiashokananda.com.

Overview of the Exercises

A coloured lotus above each exercise indicates its level of difficulty.

Posture

If you find it very uncomfortable to sit on the floor cross-legged or in vajrasana (see page 87), try using a chair. If you are seated cross-legged, keep your hips a little higher than your knees to maintain good blood circulation. Don't slouch (support your back if you need to). Your spine should be aligned, with a slight sense of elevation, from your pelvis through the front, back and side muscles of your torso. Always make sure that your spine is not compressed, to allow the flow of energy through to your head. Even if you are lying down, align your spine and have an awareness of your body fanning out from the spinal column.

Gently release your shoulders down your back and relax your diaphragm (unless it is an exercise where you are actively inhaling and exhaling with force). Unless instructed to do otherwise, keep the muscles of your head (especially in your face and forehead) relaxed. Keep your eyeballs soft behind your closed eyelids. You should not feel any lightheadedness or strain in your sinuses.

When you are ready to get up from a lying position, roll over onto your left side using your left hand as a pillow, and position your right hand ready to lend support from the floor. Pause for a couple of breaths, then push into your right hand and come up to any comfortable sitting posture.

Meditation practice may bring up feelings of discomfort, resistance, irritation or unease. This is usually the result of deep-rooted emotions that are coming up to the surface to be released either physically or emotionally. The release may take place after a few days of practising and is completely normal. You may find that you go through three stages in your journey toward transcendence:

1 **Senses**: Your mind becomes aware of a sense of non-attachment to certain things to which it was previously attached, or desired or thought it needed.

2 **Subtle body and psychology**: You awaken to chitta vrittis (chitta is your consciousness, and vrittis are the disturbances, emotions, feelings and tendencies of mind that were preventing you from seeing your consciousness). In other words, you have developed an ability to see what was keeping you from your self.

3 **Pure consciousness/spirit/soul**: You have the memory of 'conscious witnessing' – in this state you can plant the seed for self-religion (swadharma) and total, pure relaxation. This is your true existence.

CHAPTER 1

The Power of You

This chapter examines what we mean by true relaxation – a state that leads to good health, happiness and increased productivity. Harnessing the energy of your subtle body and acquiring self-knowledge are key to relaxing into your true self and realizing your inner power. This chapter also looks at the traditional yogic beliefs that have influenced the techniques and practices in this book. The exercises at the end of the chapter will start you on your journey of self-discovery by encouraging self-examination, self-awareness and self-acceptance.

'We have become more intellectual but we have lost our inner wisdom and heart. We have lost our awareness. Whatever we are gaining, we are gaining at the cost of our soul.'

YOGI ASHOKANANDA

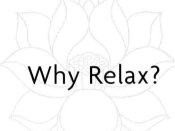

Why Relax?

Science is considered to be something that is researched, tangible and therefore generally trusted. True relaxation is a science, experienced and described by many ancient and modern-day yogis, saints and sages. It is not just about being able to rest (that is something you do when you sleep), nor is it sitting in front of the television with a stiff drink after a hard day's work. We associate meditation with relaxation, but there are also other practices that can assist in relaxing the mind and nervous system. Deep relaxation involves the interaction and engagement of body and mind. It frees you from troublesome and fragmented thoughts, memories and emotions so your mind is clear and alert, whole and complete. Relaxation can be a complete therapy which, if used regularly, keeps you in optimal health and allows you to rediscover your stillness, your silence within, your true self and your source of creation.

Many of us are overworked, overstretched and overstimulated. The world holds many threats and dangers – real and imagined – which cause us stress. We are never far from the latest news or the pressures of instant communication, reminders and updates. We are led to believe that we should be constantly setting ourselves goals and chasing exciting new experiences. We become competitive and judgmental, comparing ourselves with others and setting ourselves impossibly high standards. Mass media encourages this trend as people broadcast every event, acquisition, success (and sometimes failure) in their lives in order to attract attention to themselves.

We may fill our spare minutes and hours with recreation, but true relaxation is something we rarely make time for. Some people may even question whether inner peace and quiet are actually worthwhile because, looking from the outside, it appears as if nothing is being achieved. We think we are acting in our children's best interests by giving them the same busy, activity-filled lives that we ourselves have. We do not allow them the space to become a little bored and explore the world for themselves, and we suffocate their hidden potential by anticipating every need and making them full before they have the chance to be hungry. We overstimulate them and we do the same to ourselves. We create children in our own image rather than holding the space for them to be individuals.

Relaxation, however, is vitally important on so many levels – not only does it benefit your physical, mental and emotional health, but it also reconnects you with the still centre of your being. This is a place where you can live peacefully and happily. An overly busy mind ends up being ineffective, frustrated and stressed. While it is great to accumulate information, to be brimming with ideas and so on, a silent mind can be your most powerful tool for achieving success in the outside world. Once you have slowed down and discovered this place of stillness, you can realize and accept your areas of strength as well as any shortcomings. Having the courage to be who you are makes it much easier to tap into your creative ability and fulfil your potential.

EFFECTS OF RELAXATION ON THE NERVOUS SYSTEM

The parasympathetic nervous system (PNS) is the branch of the autonomic nervous system responsible for bringing your body back to a state of equilibrium after it has experienced a stressful situation. Purposeful activation of the PNS through relaxation has a number of benefits for the mind and body, including:

- slowing the heart rate
- lowering blood pressure
- slowing down and deepening breathing, so more oxygen reaches the cells of the body
- releasing endorphins and serotonin
- returning to normal bodily functions that have been inhibited by muscle tension (e.g. digestion, elimination of waste and production of white blood cells)
- reducing stress
- increasing positive emotions
- possibly slowing down the physical and psychological ageing processes through the effects of increased prana – your life force.

The Power of Self-realization

Many philosophers have debated the nature of the true self or spirit, but it is generally taken to mean the purest part of you, where you feel accepted, certain, safe and calm, undisturbed by the confusion and demands of the everyday self (the ego). The true self is where your wisdom, compassion and power reside, where you cannot be touched or harmed by negative thoughts and the stresses of daily living. According to Hindu philosophy, in order to achieve salvation or liberation, you must first acquire self-knowledge (atma jnana) – this is the realization that the true self (atman) is identical with the transcendent self or universal reality (Brahman). The Bhagavad Gita vividly conveys the sense of the spirit as being all-powerful, indestructible and eternal: 'Weapons cannot cut it, fire cannot burn it, water cannot wet it and wind cannot dry it, because it is still, immovable, immortal, absolute and whole.'

People often have glimpses of their true self in times of crisis or at turning points in their lives when they have to make important choices. Dreams and visions are also ways in which our higher self may try to reach us, but unless we are grounded, these imaginings can be mere distractions or fantasies that take us away from the here-and-now of who and what we are and where we really need to be going in life. If we can develop a quality of self-awareness in each moment and fully embrace our true self, we discover an invaluable source of power – a wonderful opportunity to live life to the full, infused with a sense of strength, resilience, optimism, energy, purpose, focus, compassion and creativity.

To have a sense of serenity and be able to experience the positive effects of deep relaxation on your nervous system, you must be master of your thoughts. This does not mean controlling or not controlling them or your state of mind. It is more to do with how present and how conscious of your thoughts and your mind–body connection you are. Every thought produces a reaction in your body, energetically as well as physically, and the response depends on how centred or off-centred you are. Your actions also reflect your thinking. If you can master your thinking and your activity, your experience of life will automatically alter.

It is also essential to 'surrender'. This means letting go of earthly concerns and illusion, and instead acknowledging that we are part of the universal flow. In other words, we have to surrender our individual self to an impersonal, universal consciousness. Total relaxation or surrender is only possible when the mind transcends everyday thought processes into a blissful state of pure consciousness.

The earliest references to meditative practice, often known by the generic term 'yoga', are found in the Upanishads (see page 27). 'Yoga' comes from the Sanskrit word yuj, meaning 'yoke', as yoga sought to unite or yoke the self (atman) with the universal reality (Brahman). In the West, yoga is mainly used for health and relaxation, and is associated with body postures (asanas), breath control (pranayama), gestures (mudras) and meditation. The form of yoga I teach is a holistic practice that uses all the aforementioned techniques, plus purification rituals, to regulate energy flow (prana) and align energy in the spine with the brain (kundalini). These practices also balance opposing elements and energies, such as fire and water, hot and cold, male and female, positive and negative, and consciousness (purusha) and matter (prakriti), in order to achieve higher consciousness (samadhi).

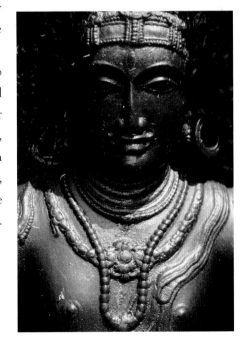

Many people are subject to stress in their everyday lives and the effect of this stress on their body's organs, immune system, and mental and emotional health are well documented. Fortunately, meditation can provide an effective way to calm the body and the mind.

Sculpture of Shiva – the Adiyogi (originator of yoga) – from the 12th-century Airavateswara temple, Darasuram, Tamil Nadu.

What Research Tells Us About Meditation

Scientific research into the benefits of meditation, as well as the evidence provided by my students and my own personal experience, all convince me that the relaxation methods I teach, based on traditional practice, are as effective and relevant today as in ancient times.

I am including here a brief survey of key scientific studies that in recent years have demonstrated the impact of different types of meditation practice on the brain and on our physical and psychological health. (If you'd like to read about the effect that the techniques and practices in this book have had on my students, take a look at their descriptions of their experiences on pages 153–5.)

Mindfulness meditation

Back in 1979 mindfulness meditation formed the basis of Jon Kabat-Zinn's stress-reduction and relaxation programme (at the University of Massachusetts Medical Center), which later became known as Mindfulness-Based Stress Reduction (MBSR). Research undertaken from 1995 to 1999 in the UK and Canada by Segal, Teasdale and Williams, and again in 2004 by Teasdale and Ma, found that Mindfulness-Based Cognitive Therapy (MBCT) approximately halved the likelihood of a recurrence of acute depression in cases where participants had three of more previous episodes.

The evidence base for mindfulness meditation has been growing in recent years, and in 2010 the UK's National Institute for Health and Clinical Excellence (NICE) guidelines recommended MBCT as the treatment of choice for recurrent depression. In 2013 researchers from the University of Wisconsin-Madison and the Institute of Biomedical Research of Barcelona found that mindfulness meditation practice changes gene expression. Molecular analysis showed reduced levels of pro-inflammatory genes and faster cortisol (stress hormone) recovery in meditators after participants in the study were subjected to a stress test in which they had to make an impromptu speech or perform mental calculations in front of an audience.

Other forms of meditation

A 2012 review of 163 studies published by the American Psychological Association concluded that Transcendental Meditation® (TM) had reduced stress and anxiety in those who practised it. Research published in the American Heart Association Journal in 2012 also showed the physiological benefits of this practice, such as a lowering of high blood pressure and a reduced risk of heart attack, stroke and death from other causes. Research published in the Archives of Internal Medicine in 2006 has even shown that TM can help to balance glucose and insulin in the blood, which can be useful in treating diabetes.

Barbara Frederikson, Professor of Psychology at the University of North Carolina, has researched the effects of 'loving-kindness' meditation (LKM), an ancient Buddhist practice that focuses on feelings of compassion and kindness. Papers published by Frederikson in 2008 and 2013 describe how LKM produces increased positive emotions and perceived social connections, reduces depression and improves physical health in meditators.

New avenues of research

Functional magnetic resonance imaging (FMRI), a technique for measuring brain activity, was used in 2011 in a study at Yale University, led by Assistant Professor of Psychiatry Judson A Brewer. The research found that people who practise meditation regularly are able to 'switch off' areas of the brain associated with daydreaming and anxiety, as well as attention deficit disorder and other psychiatric disorders, and showed that the default mode of experienced meditators was centred on the present moment rather than on troublesome thoughts. Researchers also noted increased levels of happiness.

Research published in 2013 at the University of California, San Francisco, indicated the possible anti-ageing effects of meditation, finding that the enzyme that regulates biological ageing (telomerase) increased by 40 per cent in meditators in the study. Genetic evidence of increased levels of wellbeing and reduced levels of stress in meditators was also found.

The Role of Tantra

Tantra is an authentic Indian system that covers all practices, rituals, meditations and aspects of life. Tantric techniques are relevant to the practices I teach because they engage not only the mind but also the physical body, making it easier to experience a deeper state of meditation.

The most ancient Tantric text is the Shiva Sutras, which takes the form of a conversation between the god Shiva and the goddess Shakti and includes descriptions of chakras, yogic practice and meditation. In the West, we generally associate Tantra with sex due to its assertion that sexual energy can be harnessed to achieve unity with the Divine, but it involves so much more than that.

Tantra is a powerful symbol of the unity of male and female, yin and yang, negative and positive, sun and moon, nature and spirit, mind and body, tangible and non-tangible. Western society constantly separates, classifies and labels things. The body is viewed as an object rather than as part of us or our place of existence. When you are out of synch with certain aspects of yourself, your body tends to hold on to tension. Tantra has an important role here. It allows you to be comfortable with and unite the different aspects of yourself, the material and the spiritual, the male and the female. The aim of Tantra is to become more aware of your own patterns of behaviour and to unite and be comfortable with the different sides of your nature, such as material and spiritual, male and female. Tantra helps you to function well, to have better self-awareness and to exist in harmony with yourself and everything around you.

Many people meditate at an intellectual level, but the forms of meditation I teach start in the body, not in the head. To discover your inner and outer self you must be grounded and integrated, bringing the lower three chakras (see page 31), representing rootedness, sexuality and self-confidence, into balance with the upper three chakras (see page 32), representing communication, creativity and intuition, at the place where they meet – the heart chakra, seat of the emotions.

SHIVA, SHAKTI AND THE SRI YANTRA SYMBOL

The earliest understanding of Tantra came from the example of the Indian gods Shiva and Shakti. Their unity is a source of creation and a symbol of the way of life known as Tantra, which offers you the possibility of understanding and accepting existence in all its forms. Shiva, the male principle, represents spirituality while Shakti, his female counterpart, represents materialism. Shiva stands for God and Shakti for creation. God exists in creation and creation exists in God – the two elements co-exist and this is the teaching and system of Tantra. This Tantric worldview is embodied visually in the Sri Yantra, a symbol found in both Hindu and Buddhist traditions, which represents the eternal creative principle of the universe and the union of Shiva and Shakti, male and female.

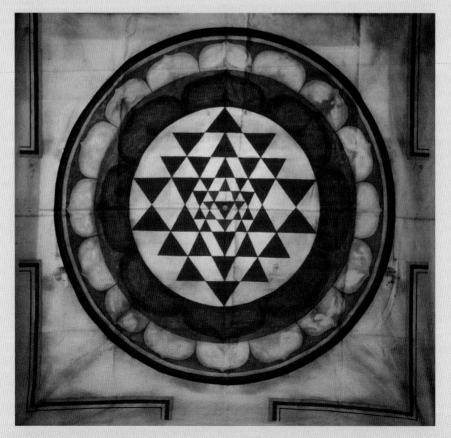

A 20th-century Sri Yantra from Kerala, representing the Tantric union of male and female. The upward-pointing triangles stand for Shiva; those pointing downward symbolize Shakti.

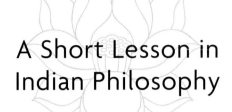

A Short Lesson in Indian Philosophy

While the practices I teach remain more than ever relevant in the 21st century, they are all grounded in traditional Indian philosophy. Below is a brief summary of some of the concepts behind the practices.

The nature of the self

In the ancient school of Indian philosophy known as Samkhya, which is based on the Upanishads, the self is seen as comprising three parts: (1) the physical body; (2) the worldly self, which includes the inner processing of thoughts, feelings and experiences; and (3) a pure, timeless consciousness known as atman, which is seen to be identical with universal, absolute truth or Brahman.

Duality

There are two basic approaches to duality in Western philosophy. In the first, philosophers hold that the non-physical self (the mind) is separate from the body although the mind and body interact; the mind determines our thoughts and emotions but is not considered the same as the living brain. In the second, only material things are thought to exist and the mind is therefore simply the brain's activity.

Samkhya argues for duality between purusha (pure consciousness) and prakriti (matter), with the mind as a refined form of matter. Whereas duality in Western philosophy is between the mind and body, duality in Samkhya is between the soul and matter. Purusha is the eternal, authentic self. All experiences and animate and inanimate objects are emanations of prakriti, which is made up of three strands (gunas): (1) activity (rajas); (2) inactivity (tamas); and (3) harmony (sattva). Due to ignorance, purusha tends to identify with emanations of prakriti such as the ego and the intellect, and this results in suffering. Liberation can only occur when purusha realizes that it is distinct from prakriti.

ANCIENT SOURCES OF KNOWLEDGE

The practices in this book come from a tradition described many hundreds of years ago in these sacred Indian texts:

The Vedas are the oldest Hindu scriptures, dating back to the second and first millennia BCE. There are four collections – the Rig-Veda, Sama Veda, Yajur Veda and Atharva Veda – containing hymns, incantations, rituals and metaphysical texts. The Gayatri Mantra (see pages 113–15) is based on a verse from the Rig-Veda.

The Upanishads are a series of Indian philosophical texts composed 1200–500 BCE, intended to be read by sages trained in meditation. They are mainly concerned with the nature of the self and teach that to understand the self is to understand everything in the universe, the single absolute reality or Brahman.

The Bhaghavad Gita is a scripture consisting of 700 verses, which forms part of the Hindu epic Mahabharata. Scholars place its date of composition between the fifth and the second centuries BCE. As well as devotional elements, it presents important concepts relating to dharma (see page 28), absolute truth and duality.

The Yoga Sutras are attributed to Patanjali in the second century BCE and comprise techniques to promote mental calmness and concentration. The eight limbs or steps of yoga include: (1) restraint (yama) – for example, non-violence, abstinence; (2) personal observances (niyama) – for example, cleanliness of mind and body; (3) postures (asanas); (4) breath control (pranayama); (5) withdrawal of attention from the senses (pratyahara); (6) concentrating on an object (dharana); (7) meditating on an object (dhyana); (8) reaching a state of oneness with the object or higher consciousness (samadhi).

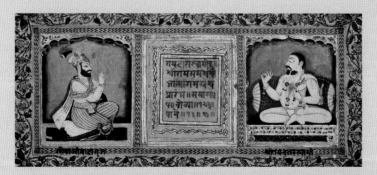

A page from an 18th-century manuscript of the Mahabharata, showing Guru Ram Das teaching the Vedas to the Maratha king Shivaji (ruled 1674–80).

In order to be released from the limitations of the physical, the self must appreciate its own pure spiritual nature. This can be done through yogic practice.

Reality and illusion

We are only able to identify objects because our senses feed us information about them. But our senses often deceive us, so our knowledge of the world is an illusion (maya). When any object is reduced to its smallest, invisible components, it is without individuality because these components are identical – this is the absolute, universal reality. Brahman cannot be known through the senses. The only way it can be grasped is by knowing our inner self (atman).

Liberation from karma

As the self is linked to the absolute, universal reality, it exists beyond the physical body and is timeless. Hindus believe in the idea of reincarnation – that when we die we are reborn (not necessarily in human form) and that this cycle of death and rebirth continues until the person has attained salvation. The circumstances of our future lives are determined according to our actions (karma) in this life – good thoughts and deeds have good effects on the next life, but bad thoughts and deeds have harmful effects. Energy and unused emotions from previous lives are stored as samskaras (see page 33) at the navel. The only way to escape the endless cycle of lives and suffering is through knowledge of atman and therefore Brahman. At this moment of transcendence, every molecule of your manifestation is freed from the memories of your karma and you are filled with the light of your awareness.

Dharma

It is difficult to translate the word 'dharma'. On a macrocosmic (universal) level it refers to cosmic order – that is, things are as they should be. Dharma is preserved by individuals living their lives in an appropriate way – through sacrifice and by doing their best to maintain optimal status quo in the social hierarchy. People also need to maintain dharma in a microcosmic (individual) way – by performing their individual dharma duty in relation to laws, customs, morals, and truth to themselves and their self-religion (swadharma).

The Subtle Body

According to yogic theory, humans have a subtle, energetic body as well as a physical form. Though anatomically different, the subtle and physical bodies are related and their balance and interplay are vital for wellbeing. Yogic practices such as asanas, pranayama, mudras, the chanting of mantras and meditating on the chakras are all used to control energy flow and equilibrium.

Prana

The concept of a universal life-force or energy is common to a number of cultures. The yogic term for this is prana (it is called chi in China and ki in Japan). Prana is all around us and is carried by the breath into the body where it circulates in channels known as nadis. Prana sustains all life forms so when the flow is obstructed, our health and vitality are adversely affected. The balance of prana in our body depends on many things including our diet and our lifestyle, our past actions and our current state of mind.

There are two main types of prana: prana (a sub-type with the same name), which circulates in the upper half of the body and is active when you breathe in; and apana, which flows downward and is responsible for elimination. For the body to function optimally, prana and apana must be balanced.

The nadis

Prana is said to flow through the body in 72,000 channels known as nadis. The central and most important nadi is sushumna, which follows the path of the spinal cord from the base of the spine to the top of the head. Two other important nadis are the ida and the pingala, which spiral around sushumna like a double helix and exit at the nostrils (ida on the left and pingala on the right). Ida is associated with female, cool, moon energy and a relaxed state, whereas pingala is associated with male, hot, sun energy and an alert state.

Kundalini energy – a powerful type of female energy – is said to lie dormant and coiled like a serpent around the base of sushumna. When kundalini is woken by yogic practice it rises, and as it passes each chakra, a different state of consciousness is reached. Along its journey, kundalini may be slowed down by granthis or knots, which prevent kundalini from rising too fast and causing physical or mental distress. When kundalini reaches its final destination at the crown chakra, the state of pure consciousness (samadhi) is realized.

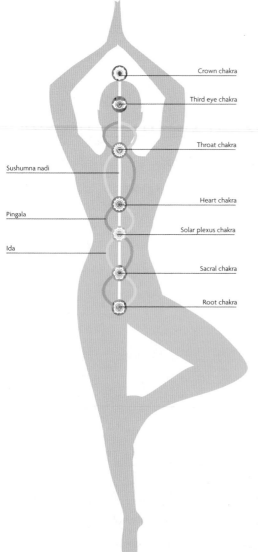

Crown chakra

Third eye chakra

Throat chakra

Sushumna nadi

Pingala

Heart chakra

Ida

Solar plexus chakra

Sacral chakra

Root chakra

The chakras

Chakras are energy centres located along the mid-line of the body. The word 'chakra' means 'wheel' in Sanskrit, and prana that passes the chakras is spun in a circular motion. Each chakra has its own characteristics and is associated with a particular element (fire, water, earth, air, ether) as well as with different senses (touch, taste, sight, smell, hearing, intuition), and specific organs, systems and functions of the body. Each chakra is depicted as a lotus flower with a particular colour and number of petals; and each chakra, and even each petal of each chakra, is also associated with a special sound.

The seven major chakras are positioned along the spine of the physical body. This is the same line taken by the sushumna nadi, the central energy channel around which the ida and pingala nadis spiral.

Root (muladhara) chakra

The root or base chakra lies below the tailbone and is where kundalini energy lies dormant. It represents the earth element and governs gravity and steadiness in the area from your knees to your feet. If your base chakra is not operating properly, you experience mood swings, insecurity and a lack of groundedness; your sense of smell is also affected and you may experience constipation (mentally as well as physically) and have a sense of heaviness in your body. In addition, because this chakra is a manifestation of individual consciousness, you lose the sense of self.

Sacral (swadisthana) chakra

The sacral or second chakra is located near the sexual organs. It represents the water element and governs the area from your knees up to your belly button. This chakra controls sex, reproduction, all activities done with your hands, your sense of taste and the activity of your body fluids. The sacral chakra is also related to creativity, the quality of your existence and your self. Any imbalance here affects your taste and your sexuality and may be related to psychological fantasy, jealousy and envy.

Solar plexus (manipura) chakra

The solar plexus or third chakra is situated in the navel area. It is influenced by the fire element and governs the area from your belly button up to your heart. It is responsible for digestion and excretion, your sight, knowledge, vigour (ojas), anger, how quickly you process and assimilate information, self-worth and self-confidence. According to yogic tradition the belly button is the centre of the body's power – the body is said to be like an earthenware pot baked by the fire of the belly. When the solar plexus chakra is balanced, the navel centre is strong and therefore the body is healthy.

Heart (anahata) chakra

The heart or fourth chakra is situated in the centre of the chest. In the Vedic tradition the heart area is known as the knot of tenderness (vishnu granthi). The heart chakra is influenced by the air element and governs the area from your heart up to your third eye (the eyebrow centre). It is where you connect your physical and emotional self with your spiritual side. It controls your heart and lungs, touch and sensuality, your relationships and attachments, likes and dislikes and your sense of joy, peace and harmony. When the heart chakra is open, you can experience true love.

Throat (vishuddha) chakra

The throat or fifth chakra is situated in the neck. It is influenced by the space (ether) element and governs the area from your third eye to the tenth gate (brahma randhra) (see page 120), where your brain divides into two halves. It is responsible for intelligence and logic, your personality, the ability to respond verbally, control over your hearing and acknowledging what you hear, and also your sense of balance. This chakra is particularly responsive to primordial sound and the chanting of mantras (see Chapter 4).

Third eye (ajna) chakra

The third eye or sixth chakra is located between the eyebrows. It represents the essence of the energy of all the other chakras, including their associated elements and qualities. Here lies the seat of your ego, the place where your intellect, intuition and judgment connect. Through the third eye you are able to begin to sense your higher consciousness and connection with the universe.

Crown (sahasrara) chakra

The crown or seventh chakra is situated at the top of the head and it is here that total awareness is achieved. Your energy and the essence of all five elements representing illusion and matter in your body are transformed as they pass through the chakras to the third eye, and meet in the crown chakra. After balancing all the chakras and the elements, and raising kundalini to this point, you are able to reach into your highest consciousness and meet your absolute truth. This is the unity of Shiva and Shakti, purusha and prakriti, matter and spirit – you are at one with the universe.

Samskaras

The cells in our body hold the memory of our experiences. Such imprints are known in the Hindu tradition as samskaras, the energetic residue of our emotional scars, and are said to be the root cause of our current emotional and physical state.

The third eye (between the eyebrows) connects via the central nervous system with the samskaras that we accumulate in our current lifetime. These are held in every cell of our body. The navel holds the samskaras from previous lives and when stimulated it acts like the mouth of a volcano from which all the samskaras (including those from this life) can explode and be released.

If samskaras are not released, they can condition negative patterns of thought and behaviour, sap energy, making us feel lethargic and depressed, and cause long-term dis-ease. For example, when we habitually hold tension within the body, the endocrine system (see pages 34–5) is forced into permanent over-activity in order to cope, which long-term can lead to ill-health.

The forms of meditation that I teach are particularly effective as they distribute the life force (prana) to create balance in the mind and body, and release samskaras. The bringing to a peak and release of a stored memory by the activation of energy flow is usually accompanied by a physical reaction, such as crying, as well as a mental realization. After release, the body and mind are connected and are able to truly relax.

It is not that we have to erase memories in order to rid ourselves of negativity – that is not part of my philosophy. Rather, it is possible to change the memories held in our mind and body and shift our perception, so that our reaction to something we once found traumatic is totally transformed.

Chakras and the
Endocrine System

The endocrine system exerts influence over the whole body by means of hormone-producing glands. Hormones are essential for the body's functioning as they regulate metabolism, growth and development, tissue function and mood.

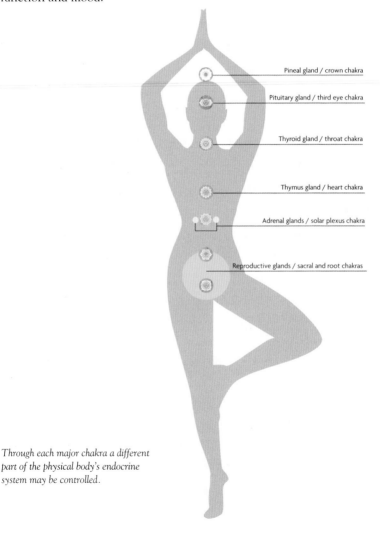

Pineal gland / crown chakra

Pituitary gland / third eye chakra

Thyroid gland / throat chakra

Thymus gland / heart chakra

Adrenal glands / solar plexus chakra

Reproductive glands / sacral and root chakras

Through each major chakra a different part of the physical body's endocrine system may be controlled.

The relaxation techniques in this book are especially powerful because they send energy directly to the areas where these important glands are situated. As each of the chakras corresponds to a principal gland (outlined below), it could be said that the physical strength and ability within our body is the manifestation of our subtle energy combined with the activation and/or pacifying effect of hormones.

The **pineal gland** at the crown chakra is sometimes known as the master gland as it influences all the other glands. It is also involved in the production of melatonin, the hormone responsible for our sleeping and waking patterns. In Indian tradition the pineal gland is said to be responsible for consciousness, psychic ability and feelings of connectedness.

The **pituitary gland** is involved with regulating the concentration of other hormones, blood pressure and growth. It also releases endorphins that reduce our perception of pain and stress. It is associated with the third eye chakra and is thereby energetically connected with memory, concentration, intelligence and thought.

The **thyroid gland** is positioned in the throat chakra and is responsible for cell metabolism and growth. Looking toward the third eye with both your eyes while lifting your chin is a quick way of stimulating the thyroid and making you feel more confident.

The **thymus gland** governs circulation and the immune system. It corresponds to the heart chakra, which is associated with emotional pain and joy. The mudra of opening the arms in surrender is said to stimulate the thymus gland, thereby improving circulation and producing a positive psychological effect.

The **adrenal glands** are situated near the kidneys and behind the solar plexus chakra. They support the kidneys (hence elimination and 'letting go') but are chiefly responsible for releasing hormones in response to stress. Energetically, this is the area of the body for drive and strong intentions; our intuition is also connected here.

The **reproductive glands** control sexual and reproductive functions in men and women and are positioned in the area of the sacral and root chakras. They are influenced by the pituitary gland.

Meditating Upon Ourselves

Swadhyana, meaning 'self-study', is a meditation from the Vedas. In traditional Hatha yoga it is known as trataka, but trataka is a substitute for this more ancient meditation. The literature describes how every morning Sri Krishna (the supreme Hindu god) meditated upon himself in swadhyana. Despite the manifestation of his energy into good and bad, light and dark, he remained in his centre.

And so it is with us today – by meditating upon ourselves, we can stay within our centre and our power. The exercises on pages 37–45 will help you to do this.

People often become obsessed with how they look – they change their appearance and adopt mannerisms that they think will make themselves seem more confident or charismatic. They assume that these things will bring them acknowledgment, care, love, acceptance and power. But neither your face value – the identity you see in the mirror – nor your self-criticism is real. They hold no meaning when you are inside your inner self. Matter is constantly changing its strength but your inner power is permanent. Inner power gives you the ability to observe change, accept it and experience life to the full.

Your mind is so active, you may find it difficult to simply meditate on your inner being or direct all your energy to your centre. In this first exercise, Face Gazing, meditating on the face connects you back to yourself.

LEVEL: ORANGE

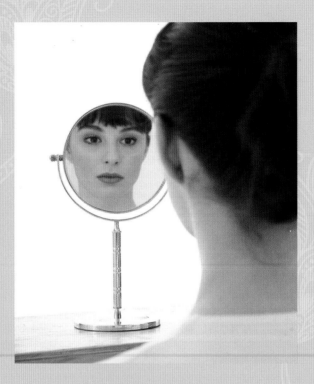

Face Gazing

The eyes are a gateway to the spirit. Gazing at your face in a mirror (known as face trataka) enables you to focus your energy to your centre and to quieten an over-active mind. This exercise will demonstrate that what you see through your eyes is not the reality – the reality is inside you. Your inner being holds the power. Everything that your senses and your mind perceive has to go back to your centre. Power is not in the object – power is inside you.

Whatever mirror you choose, make sure you only use it for this practice and not for anything else. Also, you may want to use a cushion at the end of the exercise; have one to hand if so. Before commencing, take a mouthful of cold water and hold it without swallowing while you splash your face five to seven times under a running tap. This will relax your muscles and allow prana to flow into your face. After splashing your face, stand upright and swallow the mouthful of water.

1 Sit comfortably on the floor or on a chair. Place a mirror at face height in front of you. This is your altar, where you will fall in love with yourself. Close your eyes and relax the energy of your face and your eye muscles. Relax your respiratory system and breathe normally and spontaneously. Become free from looking forward to the meditation and the idea of the meditation. Totally be with your physical body. There are only three things here: total stillness in your body, completely relaxed natural breath and your alertness. Stay with this for a few minutes.

2 Gently open your eyes. They are soft as you look at your reflection. Take in your whole face, not just a part of it. It is okay to start by looking into your eyes but make sure you widen your gaze to your whole face. Whichever way you begin this practice – either by first gazing at your eyes or first gazing at your whole face – stay with this whenever you practise and don't chop and change from one day to the next.

3 You are looking at your face as an object, gracefully, without any judgment or criticism, without liking or disliking it, without self-gratification, without calculating your self-worth, without thinking about how you appear. You are looking in such a way that it is almost as if you are stroking your face with your gaze. Simply watch the process of looking. Look in the mirror at your whole face, all in one go, with gentle eyes and without any aggression. Look for as long as you can without blinking or closing your eyes.

4 If your face starts to look blurred or appears to change shape, or if you feel disorientated, or you start seeing different people in your face, know that these are your own psychological manifestations, your own thoughts, the manifestation of the blueprint around your soul and your samskaras. Perhaps you see your spirit emerging slowly, ever so slowly, in a pure form. Do not pass any judgment on what you see and do not make any choices of liking or disliking.

5 Continue gazing at your face until it has become blurred, or you no longer identify with its features, or it disappears from your consciousness, or your eyes simply get tired. Just let your eyes close and feel the energy behind them. The flow of energy is no longer going to the outside. Just stay with this energy and its stillness.

6 With your eyes closed, meditate on the energy behind them. Focus your attention here, creating a sense of stillness with no movement of your facial muscles. If your eyes and eye socket muscles are relaxed, your face energy is relaxed. You are at ease, you are with yourself. You experience the power of seeing as if you never had eyes yet you still have the ability to see. You can see your energy, your face … you can still see everything, but without your eyes being open.

7 There will come a point where the lightness, clarity and softness in your face will slowly sink down into your heart. The deeper it gets, the more your heart chakra will expand.

8 After doing this exercise for 15 minutes, notice how you now feel the same energy as you did when your eyes were open. This is because you are aligning your physical body with your subtle body. They have the same face.

9 When you feel ready, move into a comfortable seated position on the floor (if you are not already sitting on the floor). Gently lean forward and lower your head to the floor (or rest it on a cushion). Rest in this position for 1–2 minutes (unless you have some medical condition which prevents you from doing so, in which case remain upright). This is a wonderful restorative pose.

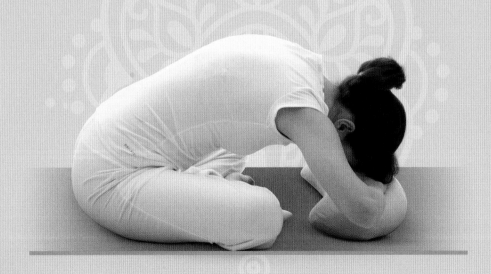

LEVEL: ORANGE

Connecting with Your Body

This exercise affects the flow of energy in your navel area, developing your confidence and creativity. It releases locked thoughts and emotions that are stuck in the vortex of your subconscious mind, brings prana to your face muscles and awakens the purpose in your life or your incarnation (avatar) in your present form. You bring prana into your body through the breath, but you cannot inhale properly until you have developed proper exhalation. Here, correct breathing harnesses the hidden strength in your belly – your internal awareness, your inner power – and brings it to your face. This exercise should be done on an empty stomach.

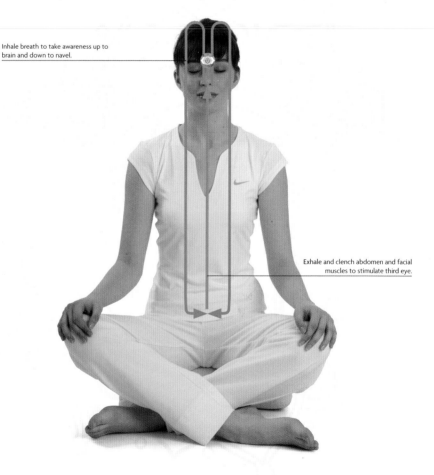

Inhale breath to take awareness up to brain and down to navel.

Exhale and clench abdomen and facial muscles to stimulate third eye.

1   Sit comfortably on the floor or on a chair. Keep your spine upright with your chin slightly raised to maintain the alignment of your spine. Place your palms over your knees. Close your eyes and bring awareness to the front and left and right sides of your brain.

2   Inhale and exhale through your nose, keeping your jaws together but without clenching them. Throughout this practice only bring physical emphasis to the exhalation. As you breathe in, connect your breath to your brain and feel your nostrils connecting to both frontal lobes. Feel your breath connecting to your navel area.

3   Exhale suddenly, squeezing the breath from your abdomen/belly button, while at the same time clenching your facial muscles so they squeeze your third eye. By squeezing your abdomen you are stimulating excretion; by squeezing your facial muscles you are engaging the pituitary and pineal glands, thereby cleansing your endocrine system and fine-tuning the balance of hormones in your body.

4   Release your facial muscles and inhale, relaxing your face and feeling the breath going into your brain. Exhale as before. Continue this exercise for 30–40 squeezes. Repeat three times.

5   When you have finished, relax and simply observe the right and left sides of your brain, your navel and your sense of peace.

✿

LEVEL: YELLOW

Rain of Energy

This meditation is good to do immediately after Face Gazing. You will find that it relaxes your whole nervous system as well as the muscles of your face and body. Using your breath, you are making your mind aware of your body and the inner space you live in, and transporting the energy of your highest existence to your lowest – you exist not only in your head but in your whole body. By engaging and connecting your third eye with your crown chakra using the breath, you are untying the knot of your karma and stimulating your creativity, bringing all your hidden powers, desires and abilities to the surface of your conscious mind.

1   Sit comfortably on the floor or on a chair. Close your eyes and keep them closed throughout the exercise. As you inhale and exhale, feel the subtlety of your breath flowing in and out and around your body. Place your attention on your third eye and feel your breath moving from your third eye to the top of your head, your crown *chakra* , as if the top has been sliced off – it may feel like you have a halo sitting there.

2   As you exhale, maintain physical energy at the top of your head – the highest part of your existence – but flush the rain of energy from this place down into the rest of your body, covering every internal and external part of it.

3   Repeat the process and stay with this exercise for around 15–20 minutes.

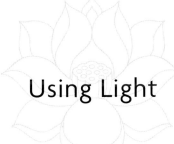

Using Light

L ight has varied and potent effects on the brain's receptors and the body's biological processes, including our sleep–waking cycle, digestion and mood. It can be incredibly healing to engage with the presence of light or even to visualize light, if you are feeling lost and disconnected from life, from yourself and from your source of power. Light reminds us of the sun, the source of all life, and gives us a feeling of lightness and brightness in the mind and body. Light also gives us a sense of optimism and even glory (Jesus, for example, is described as the 'Light of the World'). Light reminds us that we have a light within that can provide spiritual sustenance, just as in the material world the light of the sun allows the crops that feed us physically to grow.

As the light of the sun provides us with our material sustenance, so our inner light nourishes us spiritually.
Sunset in Madhya Pradesh (photograph by Yogi Ashokananda).

LEVEL: ORANGE

The Light Within

In the following meditation you use your breath to instil a sense of the powerful light inside you – your breath *is* the light – and to lessen the dark, heavy energy of a stressed mind and body. You can practise this whenever you like but it is particularly effective if you live in a country that gets little sunlight in the winter months.

1　Sit comfortably on the floor or on a chair. Close your eyes and keep them closed throughout the meditation. Breathe gently in and out through your nose. If you feel you need to release trapped energy or let go, take one full inhalation and exhale with a sigh from your mouth, then close your mouth and continue breathing in and out through your nose.

2　Stay as still as possible. Feel your body – you are not separate from it, you *are* your body. Take your whole awareness to your solar plexus or any part that you feel most connected to. Allow your senses to withdraw from the environment around you and bring them into the inner realms of your body.

3　As you connect with a point on your body, you will find that it pulsates. With each inhalation stay with the pulsation and really feel it. As you exhale, feel the light (your breath) expanding into the shape of your body. Inhaling to this same pulsation point each time and then exhaling will fill your body with warmth and radiance. Keep this image of your breath as light within the confines of your body.

4　Continue for 20 minutes, keeping a relaxed sense of the light spreading within your body as you breathe in and shrinking as you exhale. Don't try to force the images – merely allow them to be there.

5　When you have completed your meditation, take a deep breath in, gently move your fingers, toes and hands, stretch your body with a yawn and, when you feel ready, open your eyes.

LEVEL: BLUE

Light Gazing

Light Gazing (light trataka) is a more modern practice than the face trataka (see pages 37–9). Using an oil lamp as a focus helps you to develop concentration and allows your outer senses to take in the light you see and feed it back to your mind and body. (Make sure the lamp is positioned safely!) Do this exercise if you want to improve your focus and determination.

1   Sit comfortably on the floor or on a chair. Place your lamp at eye level, 24 finger spaces away, so you can just see the inside of the flame but not the lamp. Gaze gently at the flame, allowing your eyes to move around it but not away from it. Keep your facial and eye muscles soft.

2   Allow yourself to be totally in the experience of what you are doing – with your body, your face and your eyes. Continue for 20 minutes at first, increasing the time as you build up stamina through repeated practice.

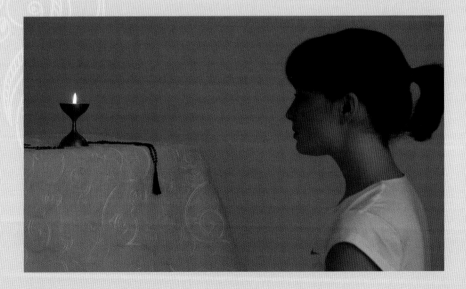

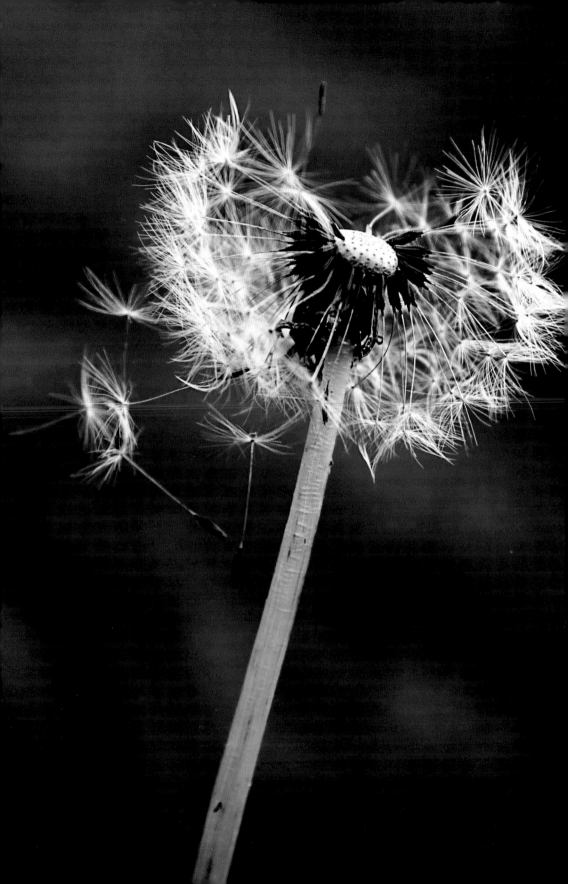

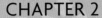

CHAPTER 2

The Power of the Breath

Fundamental to yoga and meditation practice, breath control
(pranayama) is one of the first things I teach in class. Aside from
its rejuvenating and re-energizing effects on the body, breathing
consciously helps you to make room in your mind and remain calm and
focused no matter what is happening around you. This chapter describes
the physical and psychological benefits of pranayama and introduces
you to breathing exercises that will connect you to your strong inner
self – the power within.

*'Breath is not just vital for life – it is also the bridge
between our body, our mind and our spirit.'*

YOGI ASHOKANANDA

The Importance of Breath

According to yogic tradition, the navel centre around our belly button is the source of our creation, but once we are born into the world our breath is the most fundamental part of our physical existence. Although we cannot normally see our breath, and most of the time we are not even aware of it, the functioning of our entire body and our mind depend on it.

Our breath can help us to understand the invisible, powerful force at work throughout the universe. Breath is something we share in common with every living being on earth, despite our different circumstances, different diets, different beliefs, different skin colours, different cultures, different countries, different occupations, different ethics, different paths of spirituality and so on. Whether we are rich or poor, cruel or compassionate, materialistic or spiritual, the breath is food for our spirit and we can use it to create a sense of love, peace and harmony in ourselves and among others.

Breath is not just vital for life, it is also the bridge between our body and our mind and our spirit, between matter and form and non-matter and the formless. Breath is our constant companion and is common to all living things. Yet in spite of the essential and familiar nature of our breath, few of us pay attention to our respiration unless there is a problem with it.

Learning to breathe properly, thereby boosting oxygen intake and maximizing the elimination of waste products, is one of the most powerful ways to re-energize the body, the mind and the emotions. Through the body and the mind, breath also feeds the spirit and we can use it to create a sense of love, peace and harmony within ourselves and between ourselves and other people.

Many of the imbalances that occur in our mind and body are affected and directed by our breath. It is also the case that our breath is affected by our mind, body functions, diet, posture, physical activity and environment. The breath is like a barometer, indicating our inner state, including our reactions to external

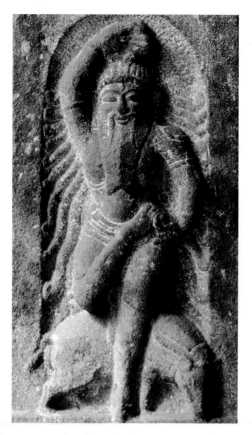

*A yogi practising breath control in Tree pose, from the medieval
Chidambaram temple, Tamil Nadu.*

events and surroundings: when we are in a tense situation we hold our breath;
when we are grief stricken or panicked we hyperventilate; when we are relaxed
and resting, our breath flows freely. The ability to connect the mind and body
with the breath and breathe naturally and evenly through *any* situation helps to
maintain a sense of calm and equilibrium in our life.

I believe that the breath has great symbolic meaning: the inability to inhale
fully represents a psychological or emotional obstruction and being unable to
exhale fully and with ease means that it is hard to 'let go'.

Any introduction to yoga, meditation or spirituality should begin with an
awareness of the breath. This is the basic building block – as essential to yogic
practice as it is to life, because the practice is there to reflect and support our life.

LEVEL: ORANGE

Meeting Your Breath

Many people spend an entire lifetime without being conscious of their breath or realizing that it is their body and mind's best friend. The following practice introduces you to your breath and calms the nervous system as well as the muscles of the face and eyes. If done for an extended period, it can lead to a very deep state of meditation and clarity of mind. It is especially good if you are very busy or suffer from stress or knee-jerk responses to events, helping you to re-engage with yourself and your environment.

1   Sit comfortably on the floor or on a chair. Close your eyes and breathe gently so you do not strain your sinuses and there is no engagement of your facial muscles as you inhale and exhale.

2   Bring your awareness to your whole body, ignoring what is happening around you or whether someone is looking at you or not.

3   Keeping your mouth closed, focus on your inhalation and exhalation and notice your breath as it moves in and out of your nose. Bring your mind's eye into your nostrils, feeling the touch of the breath on your nostril walls. As you inhale, embrace the sensation of your breath's cooling touch and freshness. As you exhale, feel your breath's warm touch inside your nostrils. Breathe comfortably for the length of your inhalation and exhalation, travelling with your breath from your nostrils to the root of your nose and back. Do not try to replicate the experience of an earlier breath or hold the memory for the next one.

4   Keep taking full breaths but slow down the speed at which you inhale and exhale, letting air enter your lungs gradually. Synchronize the speed of your breath with the awareness of your nostrils. Continue for 20 minutes.

LEVEL: GREEN

Yogic Breath

In Vedic terms the lungs represent the seat of the soul. By not using their full capacity, you restrict the amount of prana you can take in. In psychological terms this means you are not fully engaging your soul or spirit. You are literally not living life to the full! This simple exercise allows you to take a complete breath, ensuring that every part of your lungs is filled with air. Breathing fully also makes you aware of your diaphragm, helps to regulate your breath, and restores rhythm to your breathing, to your mind and to the cyclical functions of your body. When the diaphragm is tense, it constricts blood flow and tightens the muscles around it, including internal and external muscles in the back, around the lungs and especially the heart muscle. With regular practice you will gradually increase your lung capacity and feel the many benefits of breathing deeply. This exercise, which calms the nervous system and the mind, is especially good if you are stressed.

1   Sit comfortably on the floor or on a chair, keeping your spine erect and your eyes and mouth closed. Take your mind's eye to your navel centre, your belly button. Gently move your attention to your mid-chest and then to your upper chest. Just become aware of these areas of your chest, the centre of your breathing.

2   Inhale for a count of nine on one inhalation, but separate this into three parts: for a count of three inhale into the navel; then inhale for a count of three filling the lower part of your lungs; and finish with a count of three into the upper lungs and chest, filling your lungs with air right to the top near your clavicle (collar bone).

3   As soon as you have completed your inhalation, begin exhaling for a count of nine on one exhalation: first empty the top of your chest for a count of three; then the bottom of your lungs for a count of three; and finally, when you reach the navel, exhale the last of the air for a count of three.

4   Repeat this pattern for 15 minutes and notice how it induces a sense of openness, ease and release.

Pranayama

Yogic breathing exercises are known as 'pranayama', which means 'control of the prana' (see opposite). The yogic and Vedic traditions describe the practice of regulating the breath in a highly systematic way. When breathing exercises are expertly taught and practised in a traditional, holistic way, the effects are life-enhancing on every level. However, there are now many hybrids of spiritual practice, which in my view have to be approached with caution. Traditionally, techniques were taught by teachers who had many years of experience, so that despite focusing on one area, such as the breath, the rest of the body and mind would also benefit and remain balanced. I have seen many people become unbalanced physically and psychologically because the practices they are undertaking are not fully integrative. This also includes people not making adjustments in their daily habits, yet still expecting authentic results.

When I was living with my teacher, Masta Baba, back in India, at first I did not know what pranayama was. I thought that it was just the breath moving in and out, until we sat down and practised. I was literally able to see the transparency of the breath … the particles in it. I practised slowing my breath almost to the point where I felt I was not breathing at all. He made me repeat the process for many days. One day, while I was in a state of deep relaxation, all of a sudden he shouted loudly. I was shocked and gasped for breath. He told me that I had to learn to remain in the same breathing pattern no matter what. During the ensuing weeks, he would find ways to disturb me (he always knew when to catch me out!). As I continued to practise I became more and more aware of the subtlety of the mind and its connection to the breath. My mind could be so relaxed, yet the minute it was disturbed my breath reacted. My teacher explained that I must always stay with my relaxed breath, to become the breath. Eventually I discovered the power of the breath over the mind – the mind's reaction to the breath. Breath is the key to being relaxed in body and mind.

THE POWER OF PRANA

In the yogic and Vedic traditions, the breath is viewed as carrying the life force known as prana into each person's body and is considered to be the physical manifestation of this vital energy. As we breathe, prana is the inhalation and apana is the exhalation, and the time between the two is called samana. Prana is the link between the astral body and the physical body, and when prana ceases to flow, the astral body separates from the physical body, otherwise known as death.

If the flow of prana is strong, your body and brain will function well and you will be full of vitality. Your body's ability to regenerate itself will also be a lot stronger, which in turn will slow down the ageing process and any adverse effects of the environment on your body and mind.

If the flow of prana is weak, you will feel depressed, fatigued and uninspired. Anyone suffering from depression needs to be physically active (for example through yoga or brisk walking) and practise pranayama to get the energy moving. In such cases, simply sitting still in meditation without engaging in an active pranayama exercise is ineffective because insufficient prana will be activated.

Having awareness of the breath as an indicator of the functioning of your body and mind means that you can manipulate and nurture your breath to reverse or alleviate any symptoms that it is expressing.

Prana comes from the universe and its source is infinite. Pranayama enables you to control the supply of prana and influence its direction and flow in your body, bringing purification to your subtle energy system and giving you power and the ability to constantly recoup that power. Some people are more successful and influential in life than others due to the power of this prana. Every day, they unconsciously manipulate the same force that a yogi has learned to use consciously by command of his will. If you can learn to use your prana knowingly, you will never fear losing whatever you are creating. This is because you will know that your creations are controlled from a stable, powerful place within yourself, and therefore can never be lost. You become fearless because you have mastery over the manifestation of power in the universe. This is referred to as 'yogamaya', the manifestation of God's energy or creative energy, or 'kriya shakti', the power behind every action.

Breath and Space

The breath moves in space both inside and outside the body. Everything manifests in space, and space exists in everything. There is space within each inhalation and exhalation, space between each word, space between each cell, space between each molecule. Space is relaxation. Space (ether) is the biggest of the five elements in the body. Space is always required in life (for example, personal and living space, space in relationships). If we could all expand the space *within* ourselves, the world would be a more peaceful, more loving place.

People are usually drawn to practise meditation because they are feeling stressed or burnt out and are overwhelmed by the thoughts that jostle for space in their mind. Thoughts, however, are not the problem. It is natural for the mind to think, so we should not try to stop this process. What we *do* need to do is create more space in the mind and in the body, for the mind lives in the body and the body lives in the mind.

Breathing techniques and meditations allow you to experience your own inner space and to align this with the space outside you, thereby minimizing confusion and conflict within your thoughts, decision-making and personality.

THE BREATH CYCLE

We tend to think of breath as inhalation and exhalation, whereas in actual fact breath is a complete cycle joined by two invisible loops or gaps (inner breath retention and outer breath retention). The in-breath and out-breath are therefore not separate but part of one complete cycle. A practice of conscious breath retention, which is used in several of the exercises in this book, helps to balance the body's carbon levels and develops strength in the diaphragm.

LEVEL: ORANGE

Yawning

Yawning is something we all do naturally. In yogic philosophy yawning releases prana that has stopped flowing and become trapped in the body. Yawning vocally and fully is great when you need a quick boost of energy and is something you can do (almost!) anytime and anywhere.

1 Inhale deeply through the nose and open your mouth wide, allowing your jaw to release.

2 Exhale and stretch your arms up and out to the sides, making a vocal sound as you do. Keep yawning, inducing the yawn even if at first there isn't naturally one there.

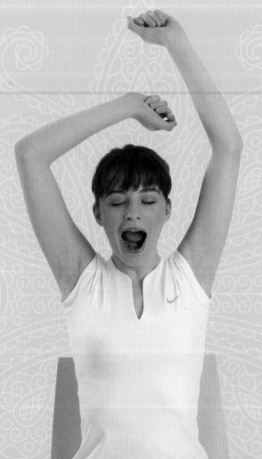

LEVEL: YELLOW

The Whole Body as a Lung

The purpose of this practice is to create more space within your body and release the obstructions that prevent you from breathing fully. You are making your mind aware of your inner space and allowing your lungs to experience inhalation and exhalation to their maximum capacity without exertion. You are also giving your mind the chance to connect and embrace the sense of oneness in your body without discrimination. As you induce a state of deeper rest through this process, you may find that your mind begins to wander. Just remain detached from whatever thoughts occur, without denying or holding onto them. Instead, only observe them and focus on the breathing practice. This exercise is good if you feel lethargic or heavy in mind and body, or if you have a tendency to overeat; you want to nourish yourself internally with breath as opposed to food.

1 Sit or lie in a comfortable position but don't use a pillow unless you really need it. If necessary, cover your body with a light blanket for warmth. Keep your heels together and allow your feet to flop outward from the heels. Relax your shoulders and your upper back. Let your palms face upward – this will help to loosen your upper back and open your heart chakra. Your arms should be at a minimum at 45 degrees from your armpits, so they are not too close to your body.

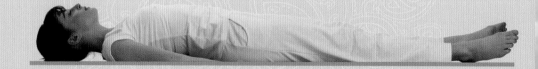

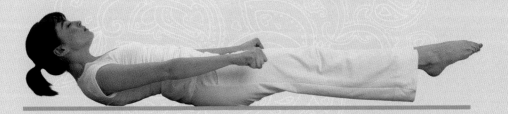

2 Squeeze your fists really tightly and release them. Now squeeze and tense your whole body, lifting your legs and your head and shoulders off the floor. Release. Repeat this three to five times.

3 As you inhale, imagine that your whole body – from your toes to your head, including your tummy, chest, ribcage and abdomen – are filled with small lungs. Divert your energy, your breath and the attention of your mind into these imaginary lungs in your body. As you inhale, your breath fills the imaginary lungs of the lower abdomen and travels all around your body, filling up one lung after another until the end of the inhalation reaches the top of the imaginary lungs in your shoulders and upper back, throat and face.

4 As you exhale, starting with the upper imaginary lungs, empty the lungs one by one all the way down, in reverse order to the inhalation. Do this as slowly and as gently as possible without any force or aggression. Practise for around 20 minutes.

5 When you have finished, relax and observe your whole body as one big lung. Feel the space inside your body all the way from your head down to your feet and fingertips. Fill your body with your mind, with your awareness; fill your body with the experience of expansion and let it go.

Breath and the Body

The Upanishads beautifully describe the interwoven physical and spiritual benefits that yogic breathing can bring. There is no separation between body and soul when physical health and balance allow full access to the spirit. This is already recognized by healthcare professionals who recommend general relaxation classes that focus on breathing patterns to help people suffering with stress, insomnia and other psycho-physiological conditions. Every yoga or meditation class should be focused around the breath.

Physiologically, when we begin to breathe properly, we simultaneously strengthen and release our diaphragm and learn to make use of our full lung capacity. Most people who are running around feeling stressed, and even those who do a lot of cardiovascular work, use only a portion of their lungs. This means that their respiratory system is not working at its best. The respiratory system fulfils two life-giving functions: to transport oxygen to every cell in the body (without which the cells would die in a few minutes) and to expel gaseous waste products, such as carbon dioxide. When you breathe fully you maximize the chances of cell rejuvenation and the elimination of impurities, and this is bound to result in a more youthful appearance and even a slowing down of the ageing process.

In addition to supplying oxygen to your body, respiration affects your consciousness, awareness and attention, which in turn are linked to mood. Breathing well can also help digestion; on the other hand, when someone is tense and stressed, the tension held in the diaphragm through constricted breathing compresses the stomach and hinders the digestive process.

Another advantage of breathing correctly is that when you inhale through your nose rather than your mouth, the air is humidified and warmed to body temperature in your nasal passages and your nasal hairs filter any impurities before the air enters your lungs.

LEVEL: YELLOW

Ujayi Breathing

The basic form of ujayi, which I teach here, is a simple technique. This ancient practice is described in the Hatha Yoga Pradipika and is commonly used in physical yoga asanas because it develops a strong heart, improves stamina, regulates blood pressure, helps with control of the diaphragm and facilitates deep cleansing. It is also excellent for asthmatics as it opens up the bronchi. 'Ujayi' means 'victorious' or 'elevation', relating to the elevation of your thoughts, your psychic ability and your heart chakra. Ujayi breathing is a nourishing, spiritual experience that burns away the darkness of your heart and clears your throat of all the unspoken emotions that affect your subconscious mind. Do this exercise to give you a more positive, lighter perception of your life.

1 Sitting comfortably on the floor or on a chair, with your eyes closed, fold your tongue backward or, if you find this difficult, press it into the roof of your mouth. (This opens the back of your throat and has a positive effect on the thymus and hence the immune system.) Inhale for a count of one, and exhale for a count of two. Regulate your inhalation and exhalation with the support of your diaphragm.

2 As you inhale with a gentle snoring sound, feel your breath touching the back of your throat.

3 With each inhalation experience in your mind the sound of 'AUMMMMMMM' (see page 109) so that your inhalation expands inside your ribcage. Try to maintain the consistency, rhythm and speed of your inhalation.

4 When you exhale, prolong the exhalation and mentally make the sound of 'MMMMM' to guide your breath.

5 Practise this exercise starting with three segments of 5 minutes and gradually build up until you are able to do a full 15 minutes without a break.

6 After practising ujayi breathing, maintain your awareness on the openness of your heart chakra, your back and the rhythm of your breath. Relax your throat muscles and breathe normally.

Breath and the Brain

You can use your breath to bring prana to every part of your brain and thereby improve your mental balance and stability. Breathing techniques can assist with concentration, memory, learning ability and being able to see tasks through from start to finish. Balancing the right and left sides of your brain aligns your thinking and creative skills. Breathing practices can even open up areas of your brain that were previously unused. Stimulating such areas of the brain helps to create a feeling of psychological balance, as well as awakening insight and bringing awareness of the ability and potential of your mind.

The breathing techniques in my meditation practices are especially good for relaxation as they allow the neocortex (the thinking part of the brain, which is responsible for analysing and judging and which tends to prevent us from entering into a meditative state) to 'switch off'. When the neocortex is dormant, this thinking part of the brain gets to rest and you can tune into the more inspired, even psychic region of the brain that under normal circumstances is hard to activate because of the busy activity of the neocortex. This is the medulla (see opposite). Often the third eye – responsible for our ego, intuition and insight – is also awoken.

When you have completed your practice, the neocortex returns to its normal activity, but the medulla will remain active, helping to counteract any mental busyness or overthinking produced by the neocortex.

LEVEL: GREEN

Stimulating the Medulla

Your breath plays a major role in controlling the flow of prana into your medulla from your spine, thereby giving you a sense of anchorage in life. This gentle exercise shows you how to use your breath safely and effectively to stimulate your medulla and awaken your psychic abilities. It will cleanse your subconscious mind and give you a sense of connection to yourself, helping you to perceive all the different parts of you.

1   Sit comfortably on the floor on a chair. Your back should be upright but retaining the natural curve in your spine. Allow your head to rest effortlessly without tilting up or down (to avoid blocking the medulla). Close your eyes and observe your breath moving in and out of your nose. Notice if one nostril feels more open than the other. Allow your breath to flow freely. Relax the muscles of your face, eyes, throat and neck.

2   Keep your attention gently on your medulla at the base of your skull, and whenever you notice your mind starting to wander, gently bring it back to this point.

3   As you inhale, allow your breath to come into your right and left nostrils and feel it travel up into the right and left frontal lobes of your brain and onward to where they cross in the back half of the brain. Your inhalation stops at the base of your skull. Keep your soft attention here at your medulla, and if your mind still wanders, keep bringing it back to this point.

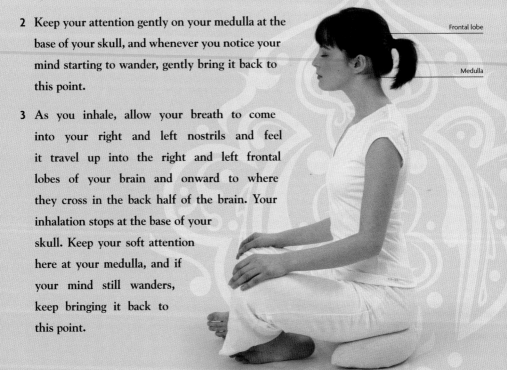

Frontal lobe

Medulla

4 Inhale and exhale into the medulla. You may notice strong images, thoughts or feelings arise. Just observe them and let them go as if you are watching a movie ... it's just a series of images going through your mind. You may also experience feelings in your body. Just be aware of them.

5 Remain with this practice for at least 20 minutes or longer if you can. When you have finished, gently rub your palms together for a few minutes to generate some energy and then place your flat palms over your heart chakra.

6 Now bring your hands over your eyes. When you are ready, open your eyes into the dark space of your palms.

7 Take a few breaths and release your hands down, smoothing the aura around your body as you brush your hands over your torso, from your back to your kidneys and hips, down your arms, and from your thighs to your feet, taking the energy down from your heart chakra to your root chakra.

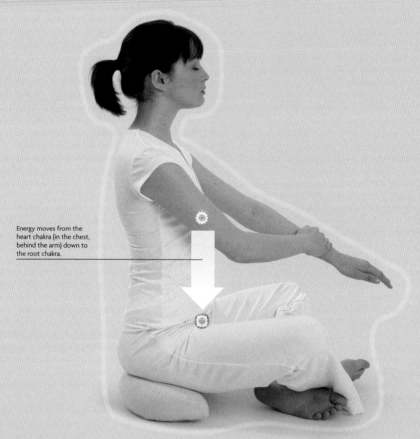

Energy moves from the heart chakra (in the chest, behind the arm) down to the root chakra.

Alternate Nostril Breathing

According to yogic thought, alternate nostril breathing profoundly affects the energetic system. It relaxes the physical nervous system, organs and muscles, encouraging an even distribution of masculine and feminine energy throughout the body and aligning the left and right sides of the brain to create coherence. This allows us to experience transparency – to perceive the source of our existence.

Our nostrils are never open equally at the same time – the flow of breath and the openness of one nostril in relation to the other changes approximately every 75 minutes. This is said to keep the brain at a healthy temperature. If you suffer from agitated, restless mental activity, alternate nostril breathing is one of the best antidotes, as this practice calms an overactive air element (vata, see page 73) in the brain. Steadying the breath enables you to calm the mental hurricane of vata, leading to a more peaceful, restful mind as well as more coherent thinking, better sleep and more assertive decision making.

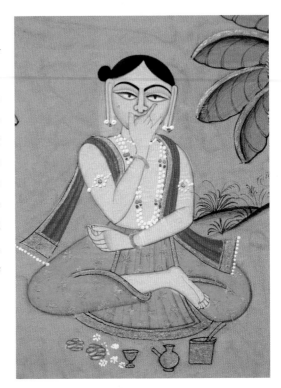

Detail from a 19th-century Indian miniature showing a yogi practising alternate nostril breathing.

LEVEL: YELLOW

Simple Alternate Nostril Breathing

This simple exercise, described as nadi shodhana ('purifying the nadis') pranayama, is often used at the end of a yoga session as it channels the prana activated during physical activity into the brain. Balancing the flow of energy to the left and right sides of the brain brings equilibrium to the mind, promotes positive thinking and optimizes mental clarity.

1 Sit comfortably on the floor or on a chair. Hold your head straight and look directly forward. For this exercise to be effective, it is important that your head is neither up nor down in order not to block the medulla (see page 61). Fold your tongue backward or, if you find this difficult, press your tongue into the roof of your mouth. (This opens the back of your throat and has a positive effect on the thymus.) Close your eyes.

2 Close whichever nostril feels the least open (you can check by exhaling). If this is your right nostril, close it with your right thumb. Apply gentle pressure on the nostril, pushing down, not across to close it. Inhale slowly through your left nostril, without straining, for as long as feels comfortable. (If you are closing your left nostril, use your right ring and middle fingers together, instead of your thumb, and inhale through your right nostril.)

3 Exhale, very, very slowly through the same nostril. You are aware of what is going on in your mind but you are observing it without trying to change or stop anything – instead you are simply allowing. You are the meditation and you feel limitless, extremely focused and very content. Your breath is the reason for this – it too is limitless, consistent and content. Repeat 12 times. Your inhalation should be the same length as your exhalation.

4 After 12 breaths, ending with an exhalation, close both nostrils at the same time and pause without breathing for the same length of time it takes for one inhalation and exhalation.

5 Now close the other nostril. Inhale through your right nostril (or the left, depending on which nostril you closed initially), exhaling very slowly. Repeat 12 times.

6 After 12 breaths, ending with an exhalation, close both nostrils at the same time and pause without breathing for one complete breath (one inhalation and exhalation).

7 Now breathe through both nostrils (keeping the same regulation) for 12 breaths breathing through both nostrils at the same time.

8 When you have completed the rounds, relax your hand in your lap. Keeping your eyes closed for a few moments, notice how your right and left nostrils feel now and see if you feel a new clarity and sharpness in your mind.

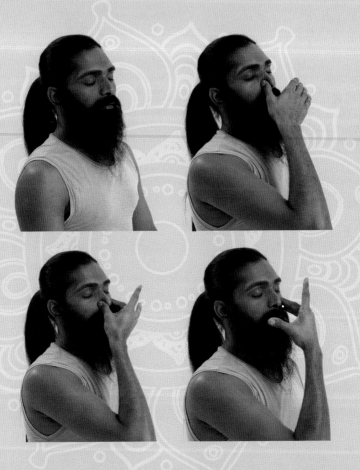

LEVEL: BLUE

Advanced Alternate Nostril Breathing

Once you are familiar with the basic technique, you can practise this more advanced nostril breathing exercise, in which the exhalation is twice as long as the inhalation. The ratio of your inhalation, exhalation and retention is 1:1:2:1. In other words, if you inhale for a count of four, you hold your breath in for a count of four, exhale for a count of eight, then pause without breathing for a count of four. You can increase the length of each segment after several months of practice, starting with a count of five for the inhalation, then six, increasing to a maximum of 16. Make sure you do not increase the lengths too early – even if one round initially feels easy, doing 12 rounds is a lot harder.

Advanced nostril breathing has a stronger effect than regular alternate nostril breathing, which is why you should do it only after having practised other exercises. It wakes up the right and left sides of the brain and stimulates the nervous system, bringing balance to mind and body.

Make sure you remain undisturbed throughout this practice. Dedicate the time to you, your healing and the experience of what is happening – from the physical to the mindful to the energetic.

1 Sit comfortably on the floor or on a chair, without twisting, arching your back or slouching. Close your eyes. Close whichever nostril is the least open, using either your right thumb for your right nostril or your right ring and middle finger together for your left nostril.

2 If your open nostril is the left nostril, exhale fully through that nostril then inhale for a count of four connecting the inhalation to a path that travels to the right side of your brain. (If the open nostril is the right nostril, connect the inhalation to a path that travels to the left side of your brain.)

3 Hold your breath inside for a count of four, connecting your awareness of holding your breath to both sides of your brain.

4 Now shift your awareness to the other side of your brain. If you have previously closed your right nostril, now close the left nostril using your right ring and

middle finger together and exhale from the left side of your brain through your right nostril for a count of eight. (Or exhale from the right side of your brain through your left nostril if you started the exercise breathing through your right nostril.)

5   Pause without breathing and bring your awareness to the outside in front of your nostrils for a count of four.

6   Inhale for a count of four through your right nostril toward the left side of your brain. (Or inhale through your left nostril toward the right side of the brain.)

7   Hold your breath for a count of four at the top of your brain.

8   Shift your awareness to your right brain, close your right nostril and exhale through your left nostril for a count of eight. (Or shift your awareness to your left brain, close your left nostril and exhale through your right nostril.)

9   Pause without breathing and bring your awareness to the outside in front of your nostrils for a count of four.

10   Now you have finished one round. Do 12 identical rounds, making sure that with each round you remain relaxed and aware and the ratio of inhalation, exhalation and retention does not change.

11   After the final round, remain with the top of your brain and feel the connection to your whole body. Meditate with openness, clarity and transparency on your brain and the space inside your head.

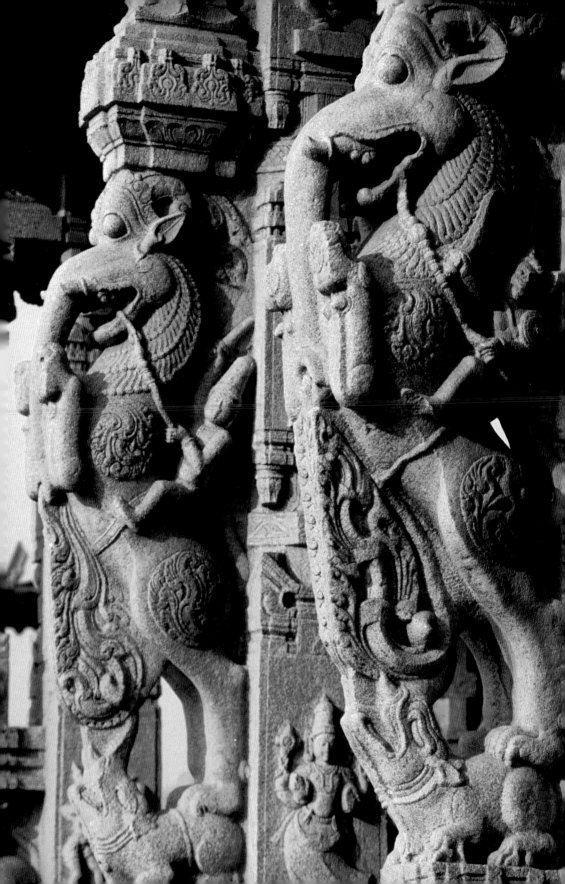

CHAPTER 3

The Strength Within the Body

Your breath, your mind and your inner power all reside within your physical form – and so the only way to achieve true relaxation is through your body. This chapter explores the mind/body connection and the relationships between your organs, your endocrine system, your chakras and the five elements. Here you will find exercises that bring you greater body awareness and stimulate energy flow wherever it is needed. As you practise, you will become balanced and centred in your self, your mind will be less easily distracted and true relaxation will become possible for you.

'Without engaging the vehicle you cannot make any journey.'

YOGI ASHOKANANDA

Why Engage the Body?

Many people who want to become more 'spiritual' or 'godly' feel that the ideal state has nothing to do with the physical body. Yet in the ancient texts, gods, goddesses and demi-gods describe their desire to be human – to be in a body – as the most amazing thing they could experience. You already inhabit your body, so learn to be in that first. That doesn't mean becoming animalistic. Before you can experience godliness, you must become totally 'human'.

In the Indian spiritual tradition, who and what we are is an intricately interwoven matrix of our subtle, energetic body, our mind, our consciousness and our physical body. Even if we are on the most fervent spiritual journey, we cannot avoid engaging the body. We should not try to avoid the fact that it is our vehicle here on earth. And our body is more than just a vehicle; it is a beautiful and miraculous creation that is in constant dialogue with our mind and our mind's interpretation of the experiences it receives through the senses. Engaging with and understanding your body and your relationship with your environment helps to create mental and emotional stamina.

MANIFESTATION

Many people try to 'manifest' or create their own reality without raising the vibration of their body and their mind. The simple practices in this book will help you to raise your energetic vibration (altering the very vibration of your body's cells) and develop patience and self-discipline. By learning to access your true, inner self through yoga, meditation and mindfulness, you can tap into your innate power and manifest it in the world. This is very different to chasing fleeting desires and whims, which never manifest themselves.

Setting off on a journey of spirituality and self-discovery can be just as seductive, if not more so, than chasing material gratification. Many people are drawn to meditation because they want to escape, to be somewhere other than where they are now. Often they have the idea that meditation is a place of refuge in their head, but this leads to a separation between body and mind and is the very opposite of what is needed for true relaxation. Body and mind cannot exist without each other. Any imbalance in our physical body disturbs the flow of energy in our mind, and this affects our potential and our actions. Whatever path we choose in order to uncover the power of relaxation within us, our body is fundamental to that journey. We must become familiar with, accept and treat with awareness every single part of it.

The spiritual path sometimes leads to an insatiable longing that is similar to the longing experienced in the material world for bigger and better things. When you only focus on dreams and aspirations in the mind, you can get carried away by a fantasy of what it is like to live a spiritual life. But when you focus on the body as well as on the mind, you are able to experience a true and ever-present state of awareness of your deeper self. You become firmly established in the centre of yourself and are less likely to be thrown off-balance by things that happen around you. Your body and your mind are both equally responsible for blocking access to your spirit (which does not need any 'work'), so give both of them your attention.

Orchards

I plant an orchard of fragrant fruits and flowers.
When my hand reaches to pick one I find nothing.
It was just a dream.
I spend every moment of my whole life creating orchards
But I always find they are just a dream.

YOGI ASHOKANANDA

The first step in meditation

Our body holds memories (samskaras) based on the five elements (fire, water, earth, air, ether). Our senses absorb the essence of the elements in the form of sight, smell, touch and so on, and these experiences are stored in our organs. Habits or karma or behavioural patterns which have become ingrained in our personality cannot be eliminated unless we employ breathing and meditation techniques involving our body. If we try to circumvent these channels, the memories enter the subconscious and continue to exert influence so we end up having two existences and two personalities, or we create the illusion of a different reality.

Bypass is impossible – this is the matrix of karma. We cannot avoid it but we can influence and change it. We have to feel it, we have to acknowledge it, and only then through meditation can we transform and live from our deepest authentic self.

I have always believed that the first step in meditation belongs in the body, not in the head. Because we are here in human form, we are in the body, so this is where we must start. When the mind is engaged with the body and when prana in the form of the breath is moved through the chakras, meditation and relaxation become an experience rather than just an intellectual or visionary concept. We 'feel' the meditation in our body.

DISCOVERY OF THE SUBTLE BODY

According to the Vedic tradition, the body – the human frame – is described as mere earthenware 'to be baked with the flame of yoga-fire'. In ancient times, the rishis (Vedic scribes) and seers discovered that the body was much more than what we normally see with our eyes. This knowledge came to them as they meditated and entered a deep state of self-awareness. With altered perception they found the formless through the world of form: invisible energy centres, channels and fields, and an integrated web of exchange and support that constitutes the mechanics of the body. They had fathomed the unfathomable and this awakening confirmed for them the existence of God.

FOOD

Food plays a major role in our health and state of mind. If you take care of your human body, the pathway to your spirit will be clear. There is an abundance of ideas and books about how to eat, but in line with Vedic tradition I recommend an Ayurvedic approach. The word Ayurveda literally means 'the science of life'. According to this ancient, holistic system of wellbeing, each person's constitution is composed of a balance of the three vital energies known as doshas, which relate to the five elements. These doshas are vata (predominantly ether and air), pitta (predominantly fire and water) and kapha (predominantly water and earth). Someone who is vata dominant, for example, may be very light-headed and daydreamy. Our food contains certain properties that will either aggravate or pacify our particular body type, so a good sattvic or yogic diet is based on foods that will balance the particular combination of doshas within us. Some recipes, such as kitchari, are tri-doshic, or suitable for all three doshas, while other foods (such as onion and garlic) are thought to provoke excessive heat in the body, especially in the liver, and are therefore avoided except for medicinal purposes. (There are many books on this topic.) Even if you can't eat according to your dosha, I advise always choosing food that is nourishing, vegetarian ideally, grown locally, seasonal and as fresh as possible. To avoid overloading your digestive system, eat to two-thirds of your capacity and don't eat too close to bedtime.

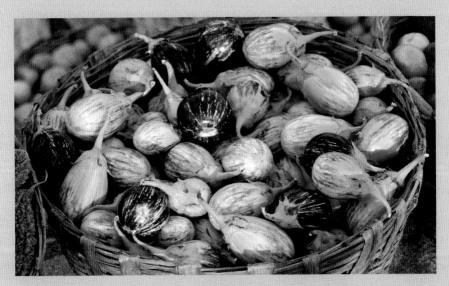

Aubergine/eggplant: its naturally stimulating (rajasic) qualities suit this vegetable to kapha types.

Balance and Equilibrium

According to Ayurveda, when we become sick we upset the whole universe – there is no separation between what goes on in our bodies and minds and what manifests itself in the world. We are all connected by spirit like beads on the thread of a necklace. This means that we each owe a responsibility to the wider world to keep ourselves in a good state of health.

Prana passes information from the organs to the central nervous system to ensure the body as a whole functions with harmony and equilibrium. Any imbalance or disturbance to the flow of prana can cause the body to malfunction. Fortunately, the correct use of the pranayama techniques and other yogic exercises in this book can correct imbalances that are creating ill-health or preventing you from attaining peace.

Imbalance in the body expresses itself in a multitude of ways, usually culminating in physical and psychological discomfort. Often the imbalance is the result of a build-up of toxins generated in the body by an unhealthy diet, lifestyle, environment or mental activity. By using my breathing and meditation techniques to gain self-awareness, it is possible to get to the root cause of such symptoms.

Acknowledging the Body (opposite) is a meditation that helps you to see that you are not the body but you are in the body. You are not there for the body but the body is there for you. Your body allows your consciousness to polish the glass through which you can see yourself and your spirit, and experience the unity of your mind and your body.

LEVEL: BLUE

Acknowledging the Body

This exercise brings your mind into your body and allows you to acknowledge and accept your own physical form. It releases muscular tension and gives you a new sense of freedom. It requires over an hour to complete: 20–25 minutes of scanning, 20 minutes of looking and at least 15–30 minutes of embracing the experience you have just gone through.

1 Lie down comfortably on your back. Close your eyes (keep them closed throughout). Let go of control over your muscles, allowing them to be as loose as possible. Place both palms on your groin area and feel the pulsation there.

2 As you inhale, scan your whole body from your head to your toes, checking if any part is tense. As you exhale, scan from your toes to your head. Is there any area where you are resisting letting go?

3 This process allows you to synchronize your mind and your body with the length of your breath. Feel your mind scanning ... try seeing your body with your attention in the middle, the front and the back. You are searching inside your body for your deepest true self. Continue scanning for 20–25 minutes until your mind becomes absolutely aware of your body and the process of the breath.

4 When you feel ready, come outside your body with your mind's eye and see your body as if it were a reflection of you lying on the floor. You are looking at your body without criticism, as if you are falling in love with your body as you look at it. Your breath is still scanning your body while your mind is outside looking at it. Your whole body looks so still and relaxed, so completely rejuvenated and energized. Your breath is flowing freely without any interference from your mind. Stay with this process for 20 minutes until you feel intuitively that your body is absolutely relaxed. It is almost as if you have bathed your body with your breath.

5 Now gently enter into your body with your mind, laying your mind on top of your body (they are the same shape and size). Observe how you are experiencing something different. Remain here for 15–30 minutes or as long as you like.

The Powerhouses of the Body

The real centres of power in the body – the chakras – lie hidden, but they can be felt through the senses and stimulated by mudras (see pages 90–93), bandhas (see pages 94–5), breathing exercises (see Chapter 2), chanting (see Chapter 4) and other practices, such as mental affirmations. Mindfully focusing attention onto a particular chakra will affect the parts of the physical body, such as organs and glands, associated with that chakra.

When you send energy to your chakras you tap into your own healing power and the ability to manifest your innermost thoughts. The energetic vibration in your body increases, and as a result your body's cells and systems respond more quickly to instructions to relax.

During a chakra meditation, energy in the form of thought, intention and breath travel up the body, activating the energy in all seven chakras from the root to the crown. When the energy has travelled back down again, the chakras are balanced energetically.

KUNDALINI ENERGY

According to the Bhagavad Gita, when we are awake, our mind is conscious and energy and spirit are in our whole body; when we are dreaming, our mind is subconscious and energy and spirit are in the back of our head; when we are in deep sleep, our mind is unconscious and energy and spirit are in our heart; but when we are in a transcendental state or within ourselves (samadhi), awareness, energy and spirit are in our spine. This is kundalini or metatron energy (also known as kundalini shakti), which awakens and rises from the base of the spine. It is our approach that determines our kundalini energy; kundalini is about awareness, not perfection.

LEVEL: GREEN

AWAKENING THE ENERGY

This 15-minute exercise promotes healing by awakening your physical body, especially the circulatory system, and stimulating the flow of energy through your subtle body. It is helpful if you have stiff shoulders and a weak upper back or if you spend a long time in a chair every day. Avoid if you suffer from high blood pressure or any heart condition, or have any major neurological or respiratory disorders.

1   Sit in hero position (vajrasana) with your buttocks on your heels. Place a cushion between your buttocks and your heels if it feels more comfortable. (If you are unable to sit on the floor, you can sit on a chair.) Keep your eyes closed throughout the practice.

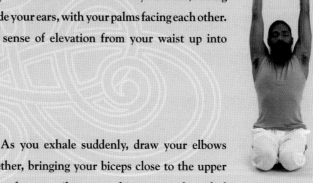

2   As you inhale, synchronize the movement of your arms, raising them up alongside your ears, with your palms facing each other. Experience the sense of elevation from your waist up into your palms.

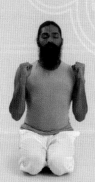

3   As you exhale suddenly, draw your elbows together, bringing your biceps close to the upper part of your ribcage, making sure they feel strong as they come toward each other. At the same time squeeze your perineum and loosely clench your fists in front of your shoulders as you lower your arms.

4 Repeat this sequence 20 times.

5 Remaining in the same position, inhale with short, sharp breaths, as if you are sniffing the breath from the front of your nostrils up to the top of your head. At the same time, throw your arms up suddenly to synchronize with your breath and simultaneously engage your perineum. It should feel as if a sudden energy is coming from your perineum and forcing you to move your arms in an excited and happy way. You should be able to feel the sensation surging through your whole body like a bolt of electricity all the way up your arms and into your fingertips.

6 Exhale very gently, with loose fists and your elbows close to your body. As you finish the exhalation you cease to move your arms.

7 Repeat this sequence 20 times. When you have completed the final round, observe your normal breathing. How did you experience the feeling of letting go?

8 For the next round, keep your perineum engaged permanently. Inhale and exhale synchronizing your sudden, active, short breaths with the movement of your arms up and down. (Use the same arm positions as before.) Do this sequence 20 times. When you have completed the final round, take some time to experience how you feel now: the flow of your breath, the openness of your heart, the sense of clarity in your head, your body awareness. Meditate upon the feelings and sensations you felt during the practice.

9 Finally, gently lean forward, take your head down to the floor, rub your hands together, and then smooth them over your face muscles, from your shoulders down to your fingertips, from your chest to your thighs, from your thighs to your feet, and from your kidneys to your hips. When you feel ready, move your legs and get up.

LEVEL: BLUE

Activating Kundalini

This chakra meditation is known as sahaj kundalini (sahaj means 'spontaneous' or 'natural'). As kundalini energy is activated and moved in a conscious way through your chakras, you begin to feel whatever is stored deep inside you and to see yourself more clearly. Engaging the root chakra will stimulate the energy to rise from this place.

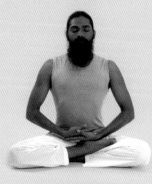

1 Sit comfortably on the floor or on a chair with your hands held palm up in samadhi mudra (see page 92). Close your eyes and take your senses and awareness inside your body. Breathe normally. Take your mind to your root chakra and as you inhale, very gently engage your anus. As you exhale, release. Continue for 50 complete breaths.

2 Take your mind up to your navel. Keep your belly soft and do 21 breaths of kapala bhati on one exhalation: that is, inhale fully and exhale sharply with short breaths from the abdomen.

3 At the end of the 21 breaths suspend your breath (kumbhaka) and create a vacuum in your belly. Hold here until it becomes uncomfortable, then release. This affects your sacral chakra and your excretory system, and gives a great sense of release. Connect with your practice, enjoy it, feel it – you are generating your own energy and can enjoy every breath.

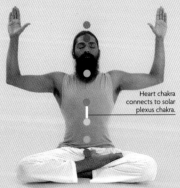

Heart chakra connects to solar plexus chakra.

4 Bring your arms out to abhaya mudra (elbows at right angles to your body and palms open). Feel the energy in your solar plexus and heart chakras and make a connection between the two. You should feel no discomfort in your chest area. Feel yourself to be in a state of not just surrender but total openness and fearlessness – a state of acceptance.

5 Be aware of the tip of your tailbone and feel the kundalini energy in your spine spinning and circling in an anti-clockwise direction and rising up. If you are ungrounded, you may feel yourself rocking slightly. Try to connect with this feeling – it is an energetic experience.

6 Inhale and as you exhale allow your breath to move from your first and second chakras and stomach through your throat. Make a gentle sound like a muffled 'mm' in your throat as you exhale. Continue inhaling and exhaling for 3 minutes, making the sound in your throat on each exhalation. After 3 minutes, feel the openness in your throat chakra.

7 Lift your chin slightly and open your eyes, looking into your eyebrow centre (shambhavi mudra). Breathe normally and remain here for a few minutes (lower your arms and rest your hands on your knees if you find the raised position too demanding).

Kundalini energy spins anti-clockwise as it rises.

8 Lie down and close your eyes. Gently engage your anus muscle. Inhale, taking your awareness to the physical presence of your buttocks and your root chakra. Forget about the rest of your body. Feel a sense of gravity here. If feelings of anger or frustration or jealousy arise, just observe these feelings. This practice will bring out anything that is being suppressed.

9 Inhale into the back of your head and then exhale from the back of your head down into your tailbone. Keep inhaling and exhaling in this way for around 5 minutes, bringing awareness to your whole spine – there is no separation between your spine and your mind or your energy. You should feel a slight tingling in your spine from the root chakra and also a sense of gentle loving care – kundalini is a very beautiful energy so treat it with tenderness.

10 When you feel ready, return to sitting or standing.

Chakras and the Mind/ Body Connection

We talk about chakras as the body's energy centres but they actually have a far wider role. The chakras are not only distributors and transmitters of pranic energy, but also inextricably linked with parts of the physical body as well as containing the five elements.

Chakras maintain the healthy relations and activities of the organs, senses, nervous system, intellect, memories and emotions. They also govern our perception and conscience and are essential for our overall sense of wellbeing.

On pages 83–5 are a series of exercises for engaging each of the chakras in turn. You can work through the whole series, to balance all your chakras, or choose to focus on individual chakras as needed.

This 18th-century Nepalese painting depicts the subtle body, including the major chakras, which lie along the spine of the physical body.

Connecting chakras, elements and body

According to the yogic system, our entire body, its organs and the function of those organs are manifested and controlled by the five elements – the five fundamental substances of fire, earth, water, air and ether. In addition, our mind is affected by every element within and around us – in fact our mind is the essence of the energy that comes out of each of the five elements. (As the whole universe and anything in it is made from the elements, these elements are alive and will therefore emit an energy.) It follows that any increase or decrease in the energy of an element causes a change in the organs and therefore alters our state of mind, nervous system and the rest of our body.

Different memories and experiences based on the elements – on what we see, smell, feel, eat and hear – are fed into the body by the senses. The chakras govern the essence of particular elements and in turn are influenced by the amount of an element's energy a particular organ uses.

CHAKRA	ELEMENT	BODY PART
Root	Earth	Colon, bones
Sacral	Water	Kidneys
Solar plexus	Fire	Liver, stomach and intestines
Heart	Air	Heart and lungs
Throat	Ether	Vocal cords, larynx
Third eye	Energy essence of all five elements = ego = mind	Head
Crown	Ether	Top of head

LEVEL: ORANGE

Engaging the Root Chakra

You can practise the root chakra exercise in isolation whenever you wish as well as at the end of a chakra meditation or of any other practice in this book. Engaging and releasing the rectum muscle while you are lying or seated stimulates the energy of the root chakra. (Incidentally, gazing at the tip of the nose has a similar effect.) Stimulating your root chakra helps to make you feel grounded in yourself and in your life. It is especially useful if you are going through a time of loss or change and are experiencing lightheadedness, or you feel like running away from things.

1 Lie down comfortably on your back and close your eyes. Counting down from 100 to zero, gently squeeze your anus and buttock muscles on an inhalation and release them on an exhalation. One inhalation and exhalation complete one round and one count.

2 If you find you lose your place, start again. Try to keep a soft focus on your inhalation and exhalation while counting down.

Engaging the Sacral Chakra

Placing attention on your sacral chakra creates a sense of free flow in your life as well as boosting your creativity and your beauty, charm and sexuality.

1 Sit on the floor or on a chair, or lie comfortably. Exhale fully, suspending your breath outside your body, without engaging your diaphragm – just allow the area below your belly button to lift naturally and connect your mind with that area.

2 Inhale, then exhale with short, sudden movements of the lower abdomen below your belly button – work up to 30 instalments in the one exhalation.

Engaging the Solar Plexus Chakra

Place attention on the solar plexus chakra to support your intention, drive and intuition. You can also work on your inner fire, which can be destructive or transformative.

1 Sit on the floor or on a chair, or lie comfortably. Inhale and completely exhale. Now move your tummy rapidly in and out without taking any breaths. Do this as many times as you can without gasping for breath.

2 Breathe in, exhale completely, pause without breathing and pull your diaphragm in as far as possible. Draw your chin into your throat and gently massage your diaphragm with your fingers.

3 Place your right palm over your solar plexus just below the sternum and move it anti-clockwise. Continue for 5–7 minutes.

Engaging the Heart Chakra

Your male and female energies meet here. Through this chakra you can deal with emotions such as love, anger and hostility, and create an inner sense of harmony and peace.

1 Sit on the floor or on a chair, or lie comfortably. Rub both your palms together really well, then place them flat on your chest and feel the warmth. Feel the infinite open space at your heart chakra as any blockages melt away.

2 As you inhale, imagine and feel the sense of a flower opening in your heart chakra. When you exhale the flower closes and when you inhale it opens up.

Engaging the Throat Chakra

Work with the throat chakra if you want to improve your self-expression, be heard clearly and stand up for yourself.

1 Sit comfortably on the floor or on a chair. With your tongue folded backward, experience your breath as it passes through your neck into your back.

2 Keeping your mouth closed, tickle your tongue against the roof of your mouth.

3 As you exhale, roar like a lion, stretching your face muscles and sticking your tongue out as far as possible.

Balancing the Third Eye Chakra

The third eye chakra is concerned with your intuition and sixth sense as well as your ego, so place your attention here if you want insight and the ability to see beyond masks.

1 Sit comfortably on the floor or on a chair. Gaze into the middle of your eyebrows with your eyes open or closed. If this exercise is new to you, you may prefer to do it with your eyes open – you will soon develop the ability to do it with eyes closed.

2 Rub your right ring or middle finger in an anti-clockwise circular direction over your third eye.

Engaging the Crown Chakra

By working with the crown chakra, you gain a sense of the ethereal and of connectedness to your divine nature, and even insight into absolute truth.

1 Stand up straight, feet slightly apart, with your weight equally distributed in your right and left feet across the front and back of your heels. Your palms are open and facing slightly forward, and your chin is slightly tilted up. Raise your left hand and let it hover 5 mm (¼ in) above the top of your head. Move it in a circular direction until you feel the vibration on top of your head or until your mind is fully established on this area at the top of your head.

2 Short and sudden inhalation is another way of directing energy and affecting the top of your head (it feels like you are breathing toward the top of your head).

3 Breathing gently, keep still as you focus on your breath inside the top of your head without frowning. Your awareness connects you through your feet to the floor and through the top of your head to the space above.

LEVEL: YELLOW

Balancing Ida and Pingala

Many people who practise meditation believe in taking the lower energy from the base chakra up into the crown chakra; they want to become connected to higher realities. While it is certainly possible to take lower energy up into the crown chakra in this way, if you do not bring the energy back down into the body, on a purely energetic and commonsense level you will be ungrounded. 'Away with the fairies' is a term that we've all heard! Daydreaming, being unable to concentrate – these are symptoms of this type of energy that is stuck up in the head and not distributed evenly through the lower chakras. When the lower chakras are energized, we can engage more fully through the senses with the physical world around us.

It's important to note that the energy of different chakras is not the same. Root chakra energy is very dense and hard compared to the higher-vibration energy of the upper chakras. It's therefore much easier to bring the higher energies down to transform the lower energies than to try to do the reverse.

When the two important energy channels ida and pingala are balanced in this exercise, an even flow of energy to the right and left hemispheres of the brain allows the third eye to open and your mind enters into sushumna nadi, the central nadi (see pages 29–30). Energy of the highest vibration at the crown chakra can then enter into the body and flow down toward the root chakra. The pineal gland is also activated, which in turn affects the flow of energy from the top of the spine all the way down to the tailbone.

The tender spots in your armpits that you press in this exercise also regulate the flow of your emotions and the left and right sides of your brain, arousing kundalini shakti.

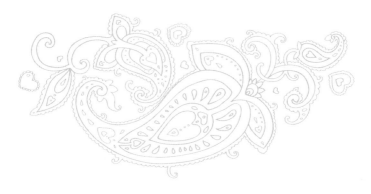

1 Sit in hero position (vajrasana) with your buttocks on your heels and your hands in brahma mudra (make a tight fist in your lap with your knuckles facing each other, see page 93). If you like, you can place a cushion between your buttocks and your heels.

2 Place your hands in hastha mudra. (This is where your thumbs press into a tender spot in the armpit – feel around a little and you will soon find the place. Extend your elbows outward at right angles to your body, with your palms facing down.) This activates the ida and pingala nadis.

3 Keep your eyes closed, fold your tongue backward and breathe through the back of your throat using ujayi breathing (see page 59).

4 Inhale once for a count of four, hold for four and then exhale for eight counts. Repeat this eight times. Do not hurry your breathing, and make sure that the force of your inhalation and exhalation is the same.

5 Place your hands in brahma mudra again. This symbolizes the connection with the source of your creation.

6 Keep your tongue folded backward, and make a snoring type of sound as you breathe in and out. Inhale once for a count of four, hold for a count of four and exhale for a count of eight. Repeat this eight times.

LEVEL: ORANGE

Enlivening the Elements

This practice stimulates all the nerves in your hands and helps to awaken all the five elements in your body, each element represented by one of the five fingers of each hand. As hands are an extension of our heart, do this exercise if you feel you need to release any tension held in your heart, any hostility or any feelings of being closed. Retaining your breath in this exercise also improves cardiovascular function, increases lung capacity and allows more carbon dioxide to be released from the body. The rotation of your arms opens up the chest, massaging the sternum, the heart muscle and the lungs and engaging your heart chakra. This exercise can also stimulate and release the samskaras at your navel and connect you with your lower three chakras, thereby keeping you grounded in your body and in your life.

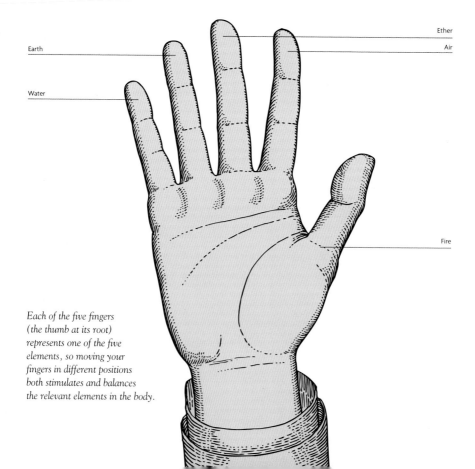

Each of the five fingers (the thumb at its root) represents one of the five elements, so moving your fingers in different positions both stimulates and balances the relevant elements in the body.

1 Sit comfortably on the floor or on a chair. Inhale, hold your breath and clap your hands ecstatically – do this quite hard (go mad!).

2 When you can no longer hold your breath, exhale and stop suddenly, then breathe normally for one or two few breaths. Experience the sensations and heat you have generated in your body.

3 Inhale deeply, retaining your breath. Allow your arms to circle and swing, and then when you can no longer hold your breath in and are about to exhale, bring your palms together again with a loud clap. Keep repeating this movement for at least 4–5 minutes. (This stimulates blood flow and fills your face and upper body with vitality.)

4 Now place your palms over your heart chakra and move the energy from your heart to your face with your palms – feel the warmth and the exchange of energy from your heart to your face. Feel a sense of love and compassion for yourself. Now experience the quietness. Feel the energetic vibration that you have created through your hands. At this point in the exercise you may find yourself laughing spontaneously. Just allow your belly button to be loose and move with your laughter. Feel a sense of the healing energy in your body that is coming out of your hands.

5 You are awakening your whole body through your hands so allow yourself to feel everything that occurs, all the physical sensations and emotions. Feel the energy through the whole of your body in a heightened state of awareness.

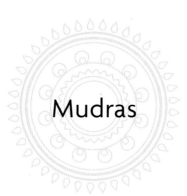

Mudras

The word 'mudra' translates as 'symbolic gesture'. A mudra is usually made using the hands, but often also involves the eyes or even the whole body. Mudras have been part of spiritual ritual in different religions throughout history. Many yogic and Tantric practices are incomplete and ineffective without them. Indeed, I have never come across a depiction in art or the sacred texts of a saint, a spiritual person or an incarnation of God in Buddhism, Judaism, Hinduism or Christianity who doesn't express some sort of mudra. Their mudra is a representation of their message – for example, authority, kindness, power, compassion, surrender, blessing or invitation.

Mudras are not just symbolic – they have a practical application as well. I once had a teacher who explained to me in depth that through the mudras you can manipulate and heal each of the five elements in your body. By directing energy to a particular point in the body, mudras activate and stimulate the chakra in that area, resulting in many unconscious physiological processes. Certain mudras are considered to be even more powerful than asanas and pranayama.

The following mudras are commonly used and can be highly effective whenever you feel you need to balance or direct energy to any particular part of your body or mind. The great thing about these mudras is that you can use them at any time, in any situation, wearing any clothes – for example, the samadhi mudra is great to do before a meeting or whenever you are feeling nervous about doing something.

LEVEL: ORANGE

Namaskar mudra

Many people are familiar with this mudra as it is a common form of greeting in India. It translates as 'saluting the divinity that exists in you'. By bringing your hands together in front of your chest, you are drawing energy to your heart but also protecting it. The mudra indicates that the gateway to God is in your heart and that this is the most vulnerable part of you.

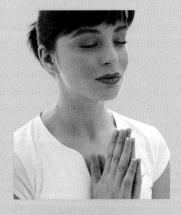

Samarpan mudra

Placing your palms flat to your heart chakra brings a sense of devotion, of surrendering to yourself and of acknowledging the sense of softness in your heart chakra. Use this mudra for paying attention to your heart, for inner reflection and for gratitude.

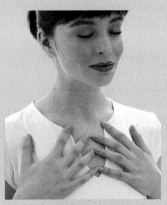

Nasikagra mudra

Looking at the tip of your nose with soft, gentle eyes, half open, half closed, engages the third eye chakra and improves concentration. It also aligns the flow of energy to your root chakra. Do this mudra when you want to focus your mind and feel grounded.

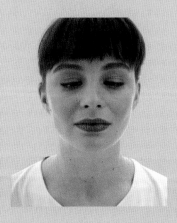

Shambhavi mudra

Looking into the place between your eyebrows activates the third eye chakra, calming the mind, awakening your intuition and providing the key to accessing your subconscious mind.

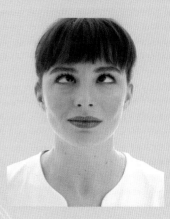

Mustik mudra

This mudra, in which your hand is held palm up with your fingers folded over your thumb, draws all the elements together in the form of your fist. It represents strength and unity within the body or that you are trying to command your mind and body to pull all the energy together.

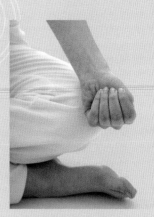

Samadhi mudra

With your palms facing upward, your right resting on your left in your lap, this mudra looks almost as if you are holding something. It shows that you are holding yourself together or that you are completely balancing the flow of energy in and out of your body to transcend to your higher consciousness.

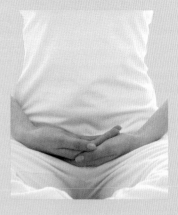

Gyana mudra

Creating a loop with your thumb and first finger, leaving the other fingers extended, relieves pressure on the brain and balances an overactive air element (vata). Too much vata makes your thoughts distracted and restless, so this mudra is good for concentration and is known as the mudra of knowledge and wisdom.

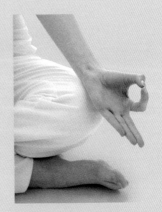

Apana mudra

Bringing the middle two fingers to meet the thumb, leaving the other two fingers extended, facilitates downward apana movement in the body and eliminates toxins. This mudra is good if you are constipated, assisting the excretory process. It also helps if you are feeling psychologically constipated, allowing the release of stuck mental energy.

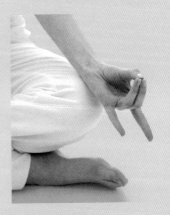

Brahma mudra

Take the tips of your thumbs to the roots of your little fingers. Close your fingers over your thumbs and press your knuckles and the front of your fingers into each other, gently pressing into your lower abdomen at the same time. This mudra is good for concentration and for bringing energy to your first granthi, the knot of creation.

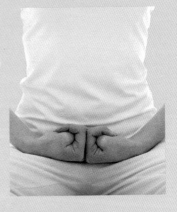

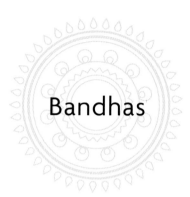

Bandhas

Bandhas, meaning 'body locks', are specific combinations of contracted muscles and are used to awaken the chakras, direct energy flow through the nadis and lock energy inside your body for detoxification and transformational healing purposes. It is thought that depictions of Christ on the crucifix may show him using mahabandha (great lock) to maintain his energy levels. Mahabandha combines three locks in one to engage the energy held in the root, solar plexus and throat chakras, as well as stimulating the associated organs.

LEVEL: ORANGE

Jalandhar Bandha

This is a chin lock that primarily benefits the thyroid and secondarily the pituitary gland. You can choose to hold the breath either after exhaling or inhaling. It is good to do first thing in the morning as part of Uddiyana Bandha (opposite), helping you to activate your powers of self-expression.

1 You can perform this exercise sitting or standing. Inhale fully or exhale fully. Take your chin to the hollow in your throat (known as 'the eternal notch').

2 Hold for as long as you feel comfortable.

3 Release, lifting your chin and curling your tongue backward as you breathe into your back.

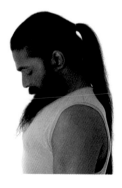

Uddiyana Bandha

This exercise strengthens your diaphragm and helps your adrenal and thyroid glands to function well. It also stimulate digestion, so try doing it in the morning on an empty stomach, after having emptied your bowels and bladder.

Make sure that you read the instructions carefully and understand them before you begin. Do not do this exercise if you have stomach ulcers.

1 Stand with your feet parallel and calf-length apart. Inhale through your nose as you squat down low, then exhale fully through your mouth making the sound 'ha', keeping your breath long and steady to the end of the exhalation.

2 After you have exhaled fully, hold your breath and apply the chin lock (see Jalandhar Bandha, opposite).

3 Press your palms on top of your thighs or on your knees and bend your knees slightly, taking all your weight into your hips. Make sure you are balanced on both feet, so you do not lean to one side, and your back is elongated.

4 Maintaining outer breath retention (holding your breath after exhaling), feel your lower abdomen being lifted upward and inward by your diaphragm. Hold for as long as you feel comfortable, so that when you release you are not gasping for breath.

5 To release, keep your chin locked, straighten your legs, relax your diaphragm, lift your chin up, curl your tongue backward and breathe into your back with ujayi breath (see page 59), through your nose only. Continue until your breath normalizes.

6 A round takes about 1 minute to complete. To benefit fully from this exercise, repeat 7–11 times every day.

The Importance of the Spine

The Bhagavad Gita states that looking at the tip of your nose while keeping your body, spine, neck and head still and straight will enable you to achieve a state of meditation and, ultimately, fearlessness.

The spine provides support for the head and trunk. The spinal cord is integral to the body's central nervous system and is connected by neural networks to every organ in the body. The spine also plays an important role in supporting the chakras and the nadis that run alongside the spinal column (ida to the left, pingala to the right and sushumna in the centre). Any blockage in the spine has an adverse effect on the spinal nerves and energy flow via the nadis to the organs, eventually causing the organs to malfunction.

Being able to connect mentally with your spine and direct energy through your spine is as important as the physical health of your spine. If the spine is compressed, physically or energetically (i.e. you have not brought your awareness to your spine), the organ corresponding to the area that is blocked will harbour stuck energy, feelings and memories and may at some point also become sick because of this imbalance. Activating the spine will affect the corresponding organs, allowing the release of energy and toxins, which will in turn send the associated memories to the brain. If the spinal vertebrae are in the correct position and aligned and blood therefore flows properly through the spine uninterrupted, so too do the energetic currents.

In osteopathy and chiropractic work, the correct alignment of the spine and skeletal system leads to the optimum health of the organs. The same principle applies to posture when sitting or lying down in meditation.

LEVEL: YELLOW

Pillar of the Body

Your spine is the pillar of your body – it supports your body and your energy centres (the chakras) and is also an integral part of your central nervous system. This meditation uses refreshing coolness and purifying heat to clear energy blockages in the spine and develop a robust nervous system. Use any time you want to give your nervous system a boost and feel more engaged with your body, if you are feeling unwell or if you are suffering from physical or mental trauma.

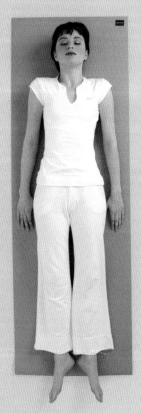

1 Lie comfortably on the floor or sit on a chair. Close your eyes, keeping them soft. Bring your whole awareness and physical experience to your back. Bring your awareness deeper into your backbone: your tailbone at the base and the rest of your spine stretching upward through your lower back, through the middle of your back, between your shoulder blades, through your neck and up to your head.

2 Inhale through both nostrils and notice a cool sensation flowing into your eyebrow centre, into the left and right sides of your brain, and then all the way down to your tailbone. Feel the breath warming up while it is inside your body.

3 Exhale from your tailbone as if you are blowing the breath through the hollowness of your spine. Feel the sense of warmth in this cavity – the pathway of kundalini or metatron. This warmth is purifying and stimulating every nerve in your spine. The exhalation is like a serpent – the eyebrow centre is the cobra's mouth, and toxins and tension are released like venom through your nostrils. When you have fully exhaled, begin the process again and continue for 10 minutes.

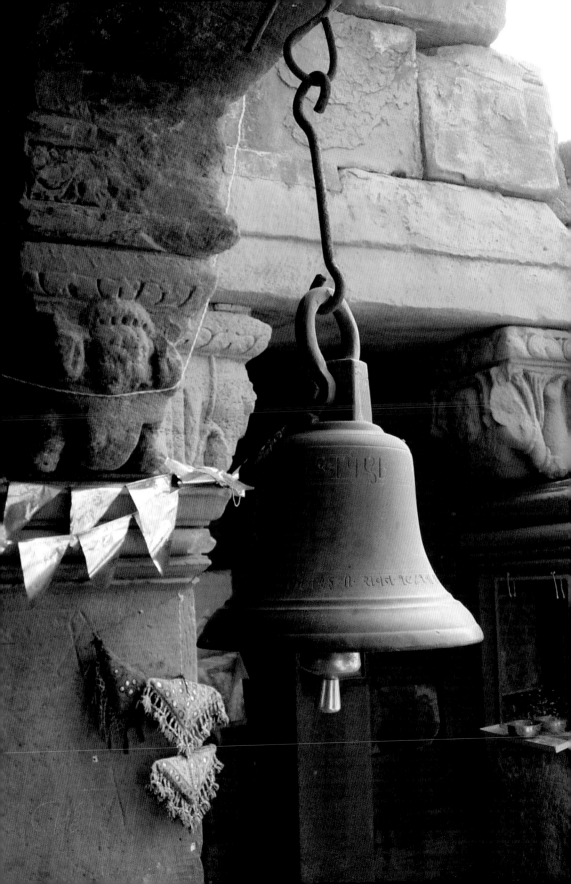

CHAPTER 4

The Power of Primordial Sound

In this chapter you will learn to use the sound or vibration of creation to stimulate and balance the centres of energy in your body. Focusing attention on the chanting of mantras calms your mind and puts you into a state of surrender in which you gain greater self-awareness. By connecting your inner voice – that is, the energetic frequency of the tiny spaces within your body – to the universal sound of creation, you can access your inner power and align it with the outer world. This alignment allows you to live out your inner light.

'By focusing on chanting, you gain awareness of yourself and reach out to the infinite source of your knowing and unknowing.'

YOGI ASHOKANANDA

What is Primordial Sound?

Primordial sound is the sound or vibration of creation, the sound that has no end, the sound that forms our mechanism, our mind and our thinking. It is all around us – an invisible frequency. Primordial sound affects the energetic frequency of our chakras and resonates with our surroundings. Every moment, the universe sounds a different note, which produces a different response and a different vibration in our brain, depending on the time of our birth. Yet when we practise primordial sound meditations, we tap into the ancient memory of our own source of creation, which ultimately is the same for us all. In this way, primordial sound reveals that we all come from the same source.

Primordial sound takes its form and expression through our individual mind and voice. In terms of helping us to find peace and power within ourselves, meditations that use primordial sound can often be more effective than other practices. This is because primordial sound is incredibly powerful in its subtle form and can quickly reach and resonate with the energetic frequencies deep inside us.

Practices using primordial sound have existed throughout history, although their form and the way primordial sound has been perceived vary in different civilizations and cultures. Mantras involve the rhythmical repetition of words or syllables to control the chattering of the mind and reach our inner well of peace and power. The mantras that feature in this chapter are said to have been adapted directly from primordial sound and contain its resonance.

Primordial sound is the instrument that switches off the neocortex, the thinking part of our brain, allowing our minds and our senses to withdraw and rest. Not only do our senses rest, they become recharged by the energy carried to them by primordial sound as it resonates through every cell in our body.

Studies have shown that babies are already attuned to vibration and sound in the womb and learn to recognize their mothers' voices even before they are born. The frequency of the universe at the time of our birth resonates with one particular chakra more than the others and thus lays the foundations for our energetic structure. Vedic astrology can ascertain your sound if you know your exact time of birth and, even if you don't know this, you can identify your particular sound simply by observing the sound that you feel most connected to or resonate with the most. I have often noticed in my classes that students who do not respond to certain practices can begin reaching into themselves as soon as chanting and sound are used, without even understanding how or why this works for them.

Using primordial sound actually awakens us on a number of levels: it taps into the source of universal intelligence that created us, it awakens our subconscious mind and the memory we had before we were born, and it has the ability to take us to deeper and higher states of consciousness – and ultimately to samadhi, the highest level of being.

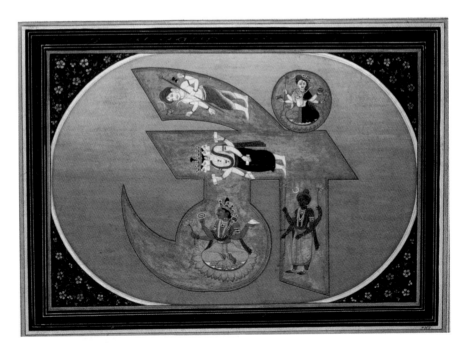

19th-century miniature depicting the sacred syllable AUM. Pronounced A – U – M, this primordial sound represents the three gunas (rajas, tamas and sattva), the strands that make up the material world.

Surrender

In this book I sometimes refer to surrendering. You can surrender to yourself or to God or the Divine. In fact, you can surrender to anything, but you must do it fully and with total alertness – be present with it and only surrender to someone (or something) who has a higher frequency than you. Something or someone who inspires you has a higher frequency than you, as does someone for whom you feel a strong, uplifting (not needy) love or who possesses holy qualities that you perceive to lift you spiritually. Often what we are recognizing in these circumstances is the higher aspect of our own consciousness lying dormant within us, ready to be awoken.

Surrendering makes you powerful as it means letting go of comparison to others, greed, feelings of inadequacy or superiority, among other things. It also means accepting yourself – at least during those times when you are trying to surrender, meditate or live a spiritual life. As long as you hold onto doubt (for example, confusion about what you believe, lack of self-confidence and trust in your intuition, or fear of losing things), there can be no total surrender. But when you totally surrender, doubt automatically disappears.

In everyday life we are not sufficiently aware of our actions – we are just intent on getting things done. We become tied to goals in the distant future instead of concentrating on what is happening in the here-and-now. We become lost in the race for wealth, social status and the accumulation of experiences and material things. We overuse our thinking brain and neglect our inner consciousness. Even in our quest for self-development, self-improvement and happiness, we forget ourselves and are unable to identify our innermost needs. To be content you need both mental alertness and self-awareness. Therefore, make your mind fully aware of what you are letting go of and surrender within your capacity.

When you focus your full attention on something (whether it is meditation or some physical task) you get to know *yourself* because you are acting with self-awareness. The use of chanting with primordial sound is one way of putting yourself into a state of surrender. By focusing on chanting, you gain awareness of yourself and reach out to the infinite source of your knowing and unknowing. The infinite source of your existence is known as viveka.

Reconnecting to Your Source

Humankind values and prioritizes scientific exploration and indeed our scientific knowledge is advancing all the time, but science is only interested in matter, not the spirit. Without self-exploration and true inner strength we are homeless, because we have moved away from our source. As the universal sound of creation, primordial sound helps us to reconnect and stay connected with our innermost self, our spirit.

Being at peace with yourself can only arise when you are free from your own samskaras. You must become aware of your own demons because until you do so, there is no possibility of self-awareness. There is no problem *per se* with improving your social status or having material possessions – these only become a problem if your way of life starts to hide your true self. Our increased understanding of the world is all well and good and can make us feel strong. Unfortunately, however, the external trappings of power can often be to the detriment of our peace, our self-awareness and our centre – they can totally displace us. Power without peace is destructive. Experiencing power *with* peace, on the other hand, is good for the development of both the individual self and of society in general. Meditation is the only way to connect to your source and bring power and peace together.

Our inner existence is pure awareness, absolute alertness, freedom from every limitation. It is self-sustained, the source of infinite power. We all have that space; we all have that power. All we have to do is look deep inside and use the tools we have to access that source.

The deeper you go, the stronger your foundations and the greater your inner strength. Your mind will become free from dense and clouded thoughts and you will become increasingly aware of your own centre. Your very existence, which emanates from that centre into your life and into society, will become the symbol of the unification of power and peace.

Primordial Sound and the Chakras

Each chakra has its own primordial sound, as does every petal of every chakra (the chakras are each represented by a lotus flower with varying numbers of petals). Together the primordial sounds of each chakra's petals affect the flow and the direction of that chakra's energy. So by using primordial sounds in meditation we can increase or decrease the flow of energy from each of our major chakras to adjust the effect of that chakra on our body. For example, if one chakra is too open and you feel that there is too much energy flowing from it, you can use primordial sound to bring it into balance with the frequency of the other chakras. You can also increase and decrease the element associated with that particular chakra (see page 82) and any emotions and feelings relating to that chakra.

Beej syllables and mantras

Beej syllables (also called 'seed syllables') are units of sound in sacred languages such as Sanskrit. Known as the sounds of the cosmos, they are universal, shared by living things through the breath that we all breathe. The syllables are used individually or together as mantras to balance the flow of chakra energy.

Beej syllables and mantras can help you to regulate your breathing if you find it difficult to breathe fully or your breath is shallow. Chanting the sound and resonance opens and relaxes the lungs at the same time and helps you to learn to lengthen your breath in a natural way. In addition, your mind is calmed because you are not using your thinking brain. You not only create more physical space in your body by opening up your lungs, but also open your mind psychologically as the expansive nature of chanting takes hold.

LEVEL: GREEN

Beej Mantras

The following mantras are normally done as a sequence. However, as with all the exercises in this book, nothing is prescriptive. If you feel stuck vocally or in a particular part of your body or any chakra, then try the appropriate mantra for that area. You can practise any one of the mantras in isolation, repeating the rounds as many times as you like. Keep your eyes closed unless you feel more comfortable with them open. Begin each of the sounds verbally to create the frequency of the sound and make your brain aware of it (afterwards you can just do it mentally and your mind will make the connection). Inhale once and as you exhale repeat the sound verbally, finishing the sound at the end of the exhalation. Inhale and as you exhale repeat the sound mentally from then on.

LAM – Beej Syllable of the Root Chakra

The frequency of this sound relates to the earth element. The root chakra has four petals, each with its own primordial sound.

Exercise: Sit or lie down comfortably. Take your awareness to the area 2.5 cm (1 in) below your tailbone. Inhale fully and gently exhale, making sure the exhalation is released evenly without forcing it. Chant LAM continuously – as many times as you can during the exhalation. Do four rounds of breathing.

Meditation: Meditate on the feelings of security, stability, foundation and steadiness.

VAM – Beej Syllable of the Sacral Chakra

The frequency of this sound relates to the water element. The sacral chakra has six petals, each with its own primordial sound.

Exercise: Inhale and exhale, repeating VAM as many times as you can manage during the exhalation. Do six rounds of breathing.

Meditation: Meditate on the feelings of charm, merging and letting go.

RAM – Beej Syllable of the Solar Plexus Chakra

The frequency of this sound relates to the fire element. The solar plexus chakra has 10 petals, each with its own primordial sound.

Exercise: Inhale and exhale, repeating RAM as many times as you can manage during the exhalation. Connect your frequency, mind and energy to your solar plexus, keeping your awareness there while you repeat the sound. When you have finished one round of chanting, observe the area of your solar plexus. Do 10 rounds of breathing.

Meditation: Meditate on the feelings of confidence, desire, will, dharma (your purpose in life) and strength.

YAM – Beej Syllable of the Heart Chakra

The frequency of this sound relates to the air element. The heart chakra has 12 petals, each with its own primordial sound.

Exercise: Inhale and exhale, repeating YAM as many times as you can manage during the exhalation. Connect your frequency, awareness and feelings to your heart as you repeat the sound. When you have finished one round of chanting, observe the area of your heart. Do 12 rounds of breathing.

Meditation: Meditate on the feelings of peace, harmony, love, unity and compassion.

HAM – Beej Syllable of the Throat Chakra

The frequency of this sound relates to the ether element. The throat chakra has 16 petals, each with its own primordial sound.

Exercise: Inhale and exhale, repeating HAM as many times as you can manage during the exhalation. Do 16 rounds of breathing.

Meditation: Meditate on the feelings of conscious self-expression, freedom and creativity and the sense of change.

AUM – Beej Syllable of the Third Eye Chakra

The frequency of this sound (sees page 109) relates to your mind and can help you with discernment, judgment and decision making. The third eye chakra has two petals, each with its own primordial sound.

Exercise: Inhale and exhale, chanting AUM as many times as you can manage during the exhalation. Do two rounds of breathing.

Meditation: Meditate on the experience of intuition, clarity, concentration, focus and discipline.

Crown Chakra

This chakra has no beej mantra. Here, observe the frequency all around your body, meditating with your pineal gland on the connection or alignment with your higher existence.

Meditation: Meditate on the thoughts of infinity, immortality and samadhi.

LEVEL: YELLOW

Vision from the Chakras

In this exercise you see and record the symbolism of each of the seven major chakras. After you have been practising for some time you will even be able to hear the chakras' energy. For a complete experience, do this exercise for 21 days for each chakra – but even doing it for one day will make a difference in your relationship with your chakras. You can do this practice as and when you feel a particular chakra needs some energy development.

1 Take some coloured pens and a writing pen and make yourself comfortable, either sitting on the floor or on a chair. Close your eyes and take your whole awareness to your root (or other) chakra without visualizing its colour.

2 Meditate for 20 minutes on this one chakra. Just breathe into it. Feel it opening up like a flower as you inhale and closing as you exhale.

3 When you open your eyes, draw and write about whatever you have seen in your mind's eye.

AUM

The use of AUM (OM) as an opening or a closing sound in yoga and meditation classes is common practice. No matter what has been going on in individual minds and lives, the chanting brings everybody together in one resonance and creates a sense of unity.

The use and symbolism of AUM is profound. The sound itself consists of three parts: A – U – M

The three parts of this primordial sound represent the three gunas: rajas, tamas and sattva (see page 26). These are the three strands – the three forces – that compose the substance of the material world.

The part of AUM that you emphasize while chanting has an effect on the granthis or energetic knots: if you linger on the A, the belly button is affected, whereas U affects the heart chakra and M influences the third eye chakra. If you wish to feel more creative or if you feel disconnected to yourself, linger on A. If you are emotionally blocked, linger on U. If you feel spiritually disconnected or are lacking in clarity, intuition or future vision, linger on M. All three parts of the sound will also liberate the three major granthis and balance energy through the solar plexus, heart and third eye chakras.

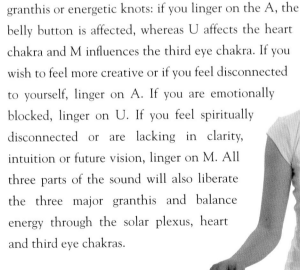

Rudra granthi

Vishnu granthi

Brahma granthi

The sound AUM influences the three major granthis (knots), which are linked to the solar plexus, heart and third eye chakras.

LEVEL: BLUE

Awakening the Primordial Sound

This exercise (available as a download from www.yogiashokananda.com) brings openness to your mind and develops the energetic field around you. If you feel depleted in energy, uninspired or depressed, this means that your aura has been blocked. Practising the primordial sound AUM will keep it open and light.

1   Sit comfortably on the floor or on a chair. Close your eyes. Inhale, directing your breath toward your root chakra. Hold your awareness here as you inhale.

2   Exhale with awareness and energy up to your crown chakra while chanting AUM four times.

3   Repeat this sequence four times. Keep your awareness at the top of your head.

4   Now inhale, directing your breath toward your sacral chakra. Hold your awareness here, then exhale with awareness and energy to your crown chakra while chanting AUM six times.

Inhale to the root chakra.

Exhale to the crown chakra.

5   Repeat for the solar plexus chakra and exhale to your crown chakra chanting AUM ten times.

6   Repeat for the heart chakra and exhale chanting AUM 12 times.

7   Repeat for the throat chakra and exhale chanting AUM 16 times.

8   Repeat for the third eye, chanting AUM twice on the exhalation.

9   When you have finished this practice, keep your eyes closed for a few minutes. Relax and stay with the frequency that you have enveloped. Feel the expansion.

LEVEL: ORANGE

Humming Bee

The vibration of this exercise is good for calming your mind, developing focus and intuition, relaxing your nervous system and increasing your stamina. Keeping your mouth closed lengthens your breath and keeps the vibration in the body for maximum impact.

1   Sit comfortably in hero position (vajrasana) with your buttocks on your heels. This generally grounding position gives you strength and directs energy into your abdomen and upper body. Place your thumbs over the flaps of your ears to close the ear canals. Using both hands, press your middle fingers above your eye bones, press your ring fingers below your eye bones, press your index fingers on your eyebrows and press your little fingers near your nostrils. Close your eyes.

2   Inhale through your nose and with your front teeth together and mouth closed hold your breath for as long as is comfortable. Feel the strength in your heart.

3   As you exhale, without opening your mouth chant AUM toward your third eye, listening to the vibration, its frequency and its sound.

4   After chanting, pause without breathing, keeping your awareness at your third eye.

5   Inhale using ujayi breathing (see page 59). Hold your breath for a short time and then exhale, repeating the chant.

6   Repeat this sequence, chanting AUM and keeping your hands in the mudra position, at least 11 times. Try to prolong the exhalation more each time.

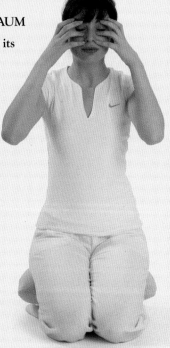

LEVEL: BLUE

Pravnav

The Bhagavad Gita refers to the practice of Pravnav. This exercise develops the ability to know or connect with your present, future and past states of mind as well as bringing together all three aspects of yourself – physical, emotional and mental. It connects you to the cosmos through your etheric body, which is your inner self. Once you are able to connect to that source, your whole physical structure and your mental state will work under your supervision, rather than dominate you.

1 Sit comfortably on the floor or on a chair. Close your eyes and notice your breathing.

2 Take your awareness to your third eye. Mentally chant AUM and let this 'sound' fill your head. Fix your attention on your third eye, keeping your mind looking internally at your brain and your crown chakra.

3 Feel the energy of the vibration from the third eye coming into your head and filling the aura around you with the sound of AUM.

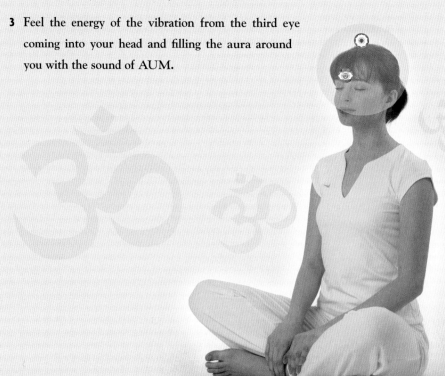

The Gayatri Mantra

The Gayatri Mantra originated in the Upanishads. It is dedicated to God in the form of the Divine Mother, Gayatri, who created the universe and bestows peace, prosperity and spiritual wellbeing. Like any mantra, the Gayatri Mantra has a strong devotional element, but this is not directed at anything outside you. It is rather about devotion to your higher self and the dormant higher energies that exist within you, and it brings with it the sense of surrender.

In the yogic tradition you are meant to inhale to the length of the Gayatri Mantra, and as you exhale you repeat the mantra in one exhalation. The Gayatri Mantra is considered to be especially powerful because it combines chakra beej mantras and primordial sounds. As striking particular keys on a piano creates a beautiful tune, so the mantra hits the right notes in the body to activate prana and the chakras. The mantra impacts on the physical and emotional aspects of those chakras, which is why you feel revitalized and cleansed after you have finished chanting it.

The Gayatri Mantra has powerful and far-reaching effects. It gives your mind access to the different dimensions of your existence, making it easier for prana to transform dead energy within every cell of your body and your brain. It enables you to use the full capacity of your lungs. This mantra also helps you to develop mental stamina and it brings tranquillity to your mind, so is useful for preventing and easing many mental health conditions (for example, panic attacks). Repeating this mantra neutralizes your thoughts so that you experience a sense of equilibrium and do not remain in confusion.

AUM BHUR BHUVA SVAHA
TAT SAVITUR VARENYAM
BHARGO DEVASYA DHIMAYI
DHIYO YO NAA PRACHODAYAAT

LEVEL: ORANGE

Chanting the Gayatri Mantra

The mantra (available as a download from www.yogiashokananda.com) is still effective if you chant it with your eyes open, but closing them removes visual distractions and allows you to retain more of your energy and internalize the experience more profoundly. When you chant it repeatedly you may feel tingling in your hands and feet or a general warming sensation all over the body. This mantra is often used at the end of a yoga practice, or at the start and close of the day as an expression of gratitude. It may also be chanted repeatedly to achieve a transformational state. A student of mine once chanted the Gayatri Mantra during a long drive on the motorway (with her eyes open of course!) to keep herself awakened and enlivened.

1 Sit comfortably, preferably on the floor, and rest your hands in your lap with your palms facing upward. Close your eyes (keep them open initially if you need to read the words to the mantra). Take a long, deep, steady inhalation.

2 As you exhale (use the same force as your inhalation), repeat the Gayatri Mantra in one breath: 'AUM BHUR BHUVA SVAHA TAT SAVITUR VARENYAM BHARGO DEVASYA DHIMAYI DHIYO YO NAA PRACHODAYAAT.' This may take some practice. Imagine that the mantra is originating from your belly.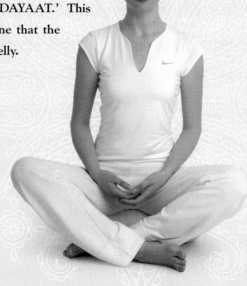

3 Repeat 108 times.

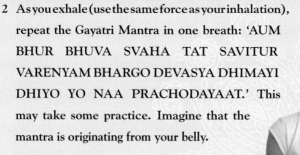

LEVEL: YELLOW

Power into the Belly

Your mind operates with the energy from your navel centre so it is important to keep the latter area strong and healthy. In this exercise you are connecting your belly and your third eye (the two main points on the body that contain samskaras) to remove any blockages in energy flow to your brain and the rest of your body. This exercise strengthens your diaphragm, releases abdominal muscle stress, prepares your body for longer pranayama techniques, such as alternate nostril breathing (pages 64–7), and releases samskaras, giving you a more spacious feeling in the body. It also takes you mentally into your body and into your navel centre so that you can be more in tune with yourself. This ability is particularly useful when certain situations in life upset you or you are about to make decisions that may not fit with who you really are or what you really want.

1 Lie down in a comfortable position. Take a long, deep, steady inhalation while mentally chanting the Gayatri Mantra, moving it into your belly button.

2 Exhale while mentally chanting the Gayatri Mantra, moving it from your belly up to your third eye. Use the same amount of force for exhalation as for inhalation.

3 Feel the pulsation of your belly button and the pulsation at your third eye as you connect these two points.

4 Listen to the frequency of your chanting but do not change or alter the pace at which you repeat it or the frequency with which you repeat it in your mind.

5 Practise this sequence for around 20 minutes, then rest for a few moments while you feel the expansion of your lungs in your diaphragm.

6 Return to sitting and observe the difference in your breath: how do you feel now when you breathe in and breathe out?

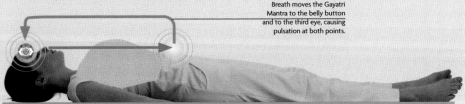

Breath moves the Gayatri Mantra to the belly button and to the third eye, causing pulsation at both points.

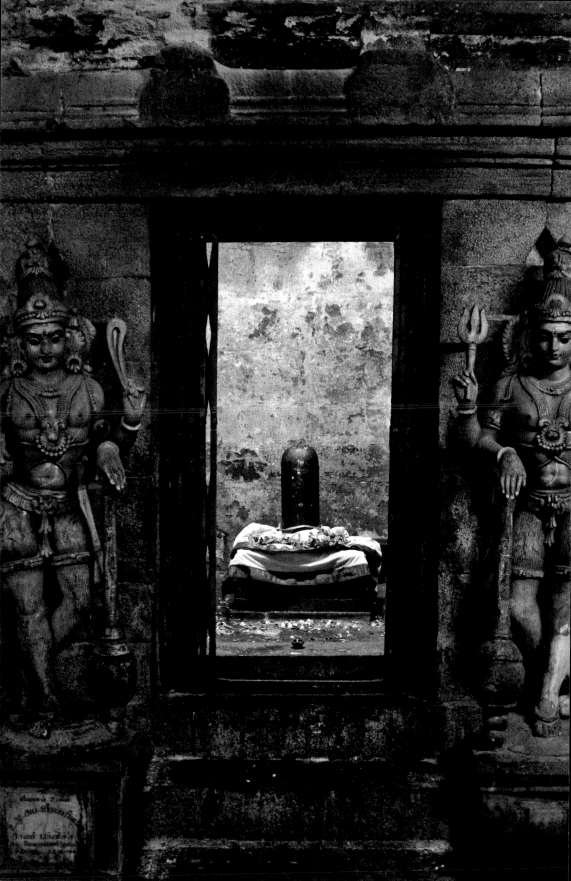

CHAPTER 5

Beyond the Duality of Life

This chapter explores the relationship between the material and the spiritual and how opposite forces are inherent in nature and our lives. To be totally at ease we need to accept our positive *and* our negative traits. We must shine the light of awareness on ourselves by going deeply into our spirit, using the pathways of our body, our physical existence and our connection to the outside world. The exercises in this chapter help you to access your inner self and to accept and balance the different sides of your personality.

'In the world most things cannot exist without their opposite.'

YOGI ASHOKANANDA

Microcosm and Macrocosm

In Vedic tradition the self comprises not only the physical body but also thoughts, feelings, senses, elements and experiences, as well as the atman (pure consciousness). According to the Vedic system, the atman is identical with the absolute reality or the source of the whole universe, Brahman. This does not mean that you take exactly the same form. The microcosm (your human nature) is made out of the same matter as the macrocosm (the universe) but it is expressed in a different way. To take the classic analogy of a clay pot: the pot is made of clay but the pot is not the clay and the clay is not the pot; rather, the pot is a manifestation of clay.

Many of us, including those who are on a spiritual path and those who are not, are conflicted by certain feelings or sensations or thoughts that exist within us. We want to be better yet we also feel pulled back by our unknown or darker energies; these opposing forces should neither be denied nor analysed in great depth. Instead, they should be acknowledged as existing because that is the nature of life and who we are.

There is a constant duality that exists on the surface level of form. Beneath this we are stillness, spirit, absolute Brahman. Our spirit is omnipotent. We are seen as separate from the universe but in reality we are absolutely bound together.

Think of the space inside and outside the clay pot – it is the same but its ability, quantity and identity differ. As long as the space stays inside the pot, it is limited. Imagine yourself as the space inside the pot. The moment the pot breaks, you are no longer; you become one with the universe and you are omnipresent. Although you have the potential to be omnipotent, you are not omnipotent because you are contained by the identity of the omnipresent. You can have the experience of being omnipresent but you cannot be omnipresent – the minute you claim omnipresence, you lose it.

Joy
In the forest of my body all the qualities exist
And the flow of joy through my veins
Increases the bliss in my heart each moment.
My heart expands with it, overwhelms with it, swirls with it.
That happiness occurs with the unity of my mind and body:
Nature and spirit,
Negative and positive,
Hate and love,
Male and female,
Uniting in love.
My awareness sings the glory of graceful unity each moment
And dances with happiness in the forest of my body.

YOGI ASHOKANANDA

LEVEL: GREEN

The Tenth Gate

This exercise helps you to develop awareness of your tenth gate (at the crown chakra), the entry point of your spirit or being, and hence an understanding of what is within you as well as outside you. This knowledge is absolute intelligence – you are connected to the universe, to God, and can experience duality without any conflict. If you are feeling mentally overloaded, try this exercise to create space and focus in your mind.

1 Sit comfortably on the floor or on a chair. Without lingering too long on any one sense, feel the space in your sense organs and the energetic quality of your senses. Feel connected to all of them throughout your body. Allow your breath to be as spontaneous and natural as possible.

2 Bring your awareness to your tenth gate (at the top of your head) and align the black hole of your individual universe to the black hole of the higher universe outside your body.

3 Remain with this practice for 20–25 minutes to feel the connection to your higher being.

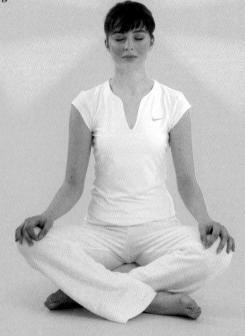

Mystery and Transparency

Life is like two river banks, with the material on one side and the spiritual on the other. You are the river and hidden deep below the surface of the water is the reality of the two banks uniting as one. The water is like maya, the mystery that creates the illusion of two. If you remove the water, there are not two, but just one. Just because you cannot see something does not mean it does not exist. Many things in the world are sometimes hidden and at other times revealed. (You only have to think of the sun disappearing from view at night as the Earth revolves on its axis around it.) You may not be able to see spirit, yet expressions of it constantly flicker in and out of your life in the form of love, inspiration, a light that switches on in someone's eyes or a child's innocence and joy.

We constantly experience the interplay of opposites in nature – for example, hot and cold, light and dark, positive and negative, male and female, acid and alkaline. Opposites have to exist in order for us to differentiate one thing from another. Without opposites nothing in the world of form would exist – light cannot exist without dark, dark cannot exist without light and there has to be contrast between objects for different shapes and colours to be seen. This interplay of mystery, form and transparency in the world is what makes life so infinitely interesting. And yet the source of this duality is one.

When we try to reach a state of true relaxation and raise our level of consciousness, we often feel obstructed by all the things that seem to be in opposition to our higher self. For example, mundane thoughts about everyday life, bodily aches and pains, emotional turmoil and external noise and distractions. For this very reason, every meditation and breathing technique I teach engages some aspect of physical existence. When we embrace what is already there and do not fight with it, we can sit deeply in the centre of our existence with peace, acceptance and surrender.

Adopting an Attitude
of Total Awareness

Almost every path to greater health or awareness or spirituality indicates that we should 'get rid of' some or other behavioural aspect or habit. Trying to do this without addressing the deep-seated root of the behaviour (in other words, the trait or karma that is locked inside us in the form of samskaras) is a temporary solution, like covering up a problem with a layer of paint. This will eventually flake off, revealing the original colour once more – just as it always was.

The breathing and meditation practices in this book are necessary for real transformation to take place. We must go deeply into our spirit using the pathways of the body in order to release the patterns that have become trapped there. The physical form is the opposite form to the spirit and it is only by embracing and working with these dualities – the material and the spiritual – that we can reach our true centre.

Duality gives us the possibility to co-exist with nature and to expand. The point is not about running away from yourself or living in a fantasy world; rather it is about staying with yourself on every level and with every aspect of your physical body as well as your emotional and psychological self. However, forcing yourself to accept a certain aspect of yourself is a recipe for failure if you do not currently feel that it is something you can accept. For this reason, I teach you first to

A fifth-century Shiva lingam from the temple at Khoh, Madhya Pradesh. The god's third eye is visible on his forehead.

shine the light of awareness on your whole self (see page 129) so that you gain a pure awareness by simply looking, before trying to accept anything in particular.

When we are distant from a light source our shadow can be large, but the closer we get to the light or if the light shines on top of us, the more our shadow creeps under our feet. Sometimes in our life we convince ourselves that through intellectual argument or analysis we have made our shadow disappear and that we are standing in the light. However, our shadow has not really gone away. If you find that your so-called shadow self or your own demons or experiences are difficult to accept, do not try to argue or reason with them, just observe and acknowledge them.

Ultimately, what is important is not the total elimination of darkness or the accumulation of the light, but the ability to experience a transparency, to see the dark, acknowledge it when we are in the light and to see the light through the dark.

THE AWAKENING PROCESS

We can only get to experience our relaxed centre of being when we accept that what occurs in our thoughts and our very nature is an expression of our humanness. This material existence and all our human feelings must be embraced in order to experience the restful yet fully powerful spirit. Brahman cannot be felt without this tangible aspect of who we are.

When you meditate with your body using the practices in this book, you will start to experience everything that it is possible for you to feel because you will be waking up your whole self. Along with this awakening come thoughts about all the things you like about yourself and your life as well as all the things you dislike. It is perfectly normal for doubts, confusion, questioning, struggles, fears and desires to appear. This is all part of your continued awakening as you journey through life. You cannot transform or heal if you do not feel all of yourself, and you will be unable to reach your centre if you try to keep only the sensations you like and repress the unpleasant ones.

Self-acceptance

Ancient texts from many traditions make reference to the world of form as illusion (maya) and to the invisible world of spirit – the life force that makes everything happen – as reality. In the past, these descriptions of the material and the spiritual life brought people an awareness of godliness and a sense of hope in times of trouble – they helped people to understand that they were part of a bigger plan. Nowadays, although the concept of illusion and reality still hold true, it seems that religion is often used to create fear and manipulate people into fighting with each other.

These concepts of illusion and reality can seem confusing, especially as we live in the world of form – we inhabit the body, we live in a physical environment and we feel the effects of that environment to a greater or lesser degree. With this in mind the techniques that I teach focus on the body, thereby embracing humanness as well as the higher self and healing any conflict or split that you may feel between the material aspects of your life and your spiritual self. Duality is like the opposite ends of a stick – two parts of the same thing. Higher awareness gained through meditation helps you to grasp the concept of duality and non-duality, and to be free from both by accepting all aspects of your existence.

You may fear that by doing this you will lose something or become disempowered. Accepting both your positive and negative traits without an awareness of your spirit is difficult (if not impossible). However, if you can be in the centre of yourself, with your spirit as your reference point, you can observe all aspects of yourself without becoming attached to any. You do not even need to avoid passing judgment – if you allow yourself to judge, accept that too.

By accepting your positive and negative traits, you end your battle with yourself – the beating yourself up in your mind for not doing this or that. Instead, you discover compassion, love and understanding for yourself and, in turn, for other people.

LEVEL: GREEN

Your Body as a Treasure Chest

This practice guides you in unlocking your hidden treasure – the inner light or energy that can dispel the fears, insecurities and dark energies that your mind has perceived. It expands your awareness, your aura and your body's magnetic field. It shines a light on all the mysteries of your mind and brings transparency to your consciousness. If you feel claustrophobic in your body, your environment or your life, this exercise will give you a sense of space. You can use it to expand your aura and it is particularly good if you are a naturally fearful person.

The exercise can take 30–45 minutes or more, so make sure you have sufficient time available to benefit fully.

1 Lie down comfortably in a dark room (use a pillow and cover your body with a blanket if you wish). Gently close your eyes. Keep your head in the south and your feet in the north. Your right side should be in the east and your left side in the west. Stretch your arms out comfortably so that they are at right angles to your body.

2 Know that your body is like a box that contains your inner space, your true self. Become aware of the inner walls of this box with your breath: firstly, take your mind or awareness to the top of your head, then to the inside soles of your feet, then to the right side of your body, then to the left side of your body, then to the top of your body and finally to the bottom of your body.

3 Bring your awareness of your external surroundings, which you feel and experience as empty space, to the inside of your body.

4 Expand your awareness to the north from your feet and go as far as your mind and your imagination allow you to feel and see. There is no limit for expansion – there is nothing in your way, no walls, no houses, no towns, just totally clear space. Only you exist. As you expand, there are no obstacles because objects do not exist, they are just a manifestation of the mind for the mind. You are expanding your energetic field, your aura; do not go beyond the boundary of this.

5 Expand to the east from your right side. Expand all along your side from your ankle all the way up to your ear – it feels as if your side has been unzipped. Again, do not go beyond the boundary of your energetic field.

6 Repeat the same expansion of your energetic field to the east from your left side. Go as far as you can but do not go beyond the boundary of your energy field.

7 Expand to the south from your head. It feels as if the energy is pouring out from the top of your head, expanding into the space in the south. Reach out to the boundaries of your mind and the expanse of your aura.

8 Now expand to the west from your right side. Expand all along your side from your ankle up to your ear and feel the light and energy and awareness coming out of your right side and expanding as far as possible in a westerly direction. Once again, stay within your energetic boundary.

9 Repeat the same expansion of your energetic field to the west from your left side. Go as far as you can but do not go beyond the boundary of your energy field.

10 Feel the energy pushing from the bottom of your body – there is no floor beneath you, you are pushing into space. Expand your aura and energy, create a boundary and stay there.

11 Expand from the top surface of your body up into space, as high as you can, growing your aura, almost as if a lid has been lifted and you are reaching up to the sky.

12 As you inhale, feel your body expanding in all six directions. As you exhale, feel your body becoming smaller and smaller until it is the size of an atom. With each complete breath keep experiencing the expansion and contraction of your body, your aura and your mind.

13 When you are ready, come out of the meditation. Remain lying down with your eyes closed and stay with the silence for a few minutes. Feel the space and release within your body but also your ability and power to emit your own radiance, which reveals to you the truth that duality is present within you.

Expansion of awareness from
your head southward

Flow of awareness from the top of your head to
the soles of your feet

Expansion of
awareness from your
right side eastward
and westward

Expansion of
awareness from your
left side eastward
and westward

Flow of awareness from the soles of your feet up your
right side and down your left side

N

Expansion of awareness from
your feet northward

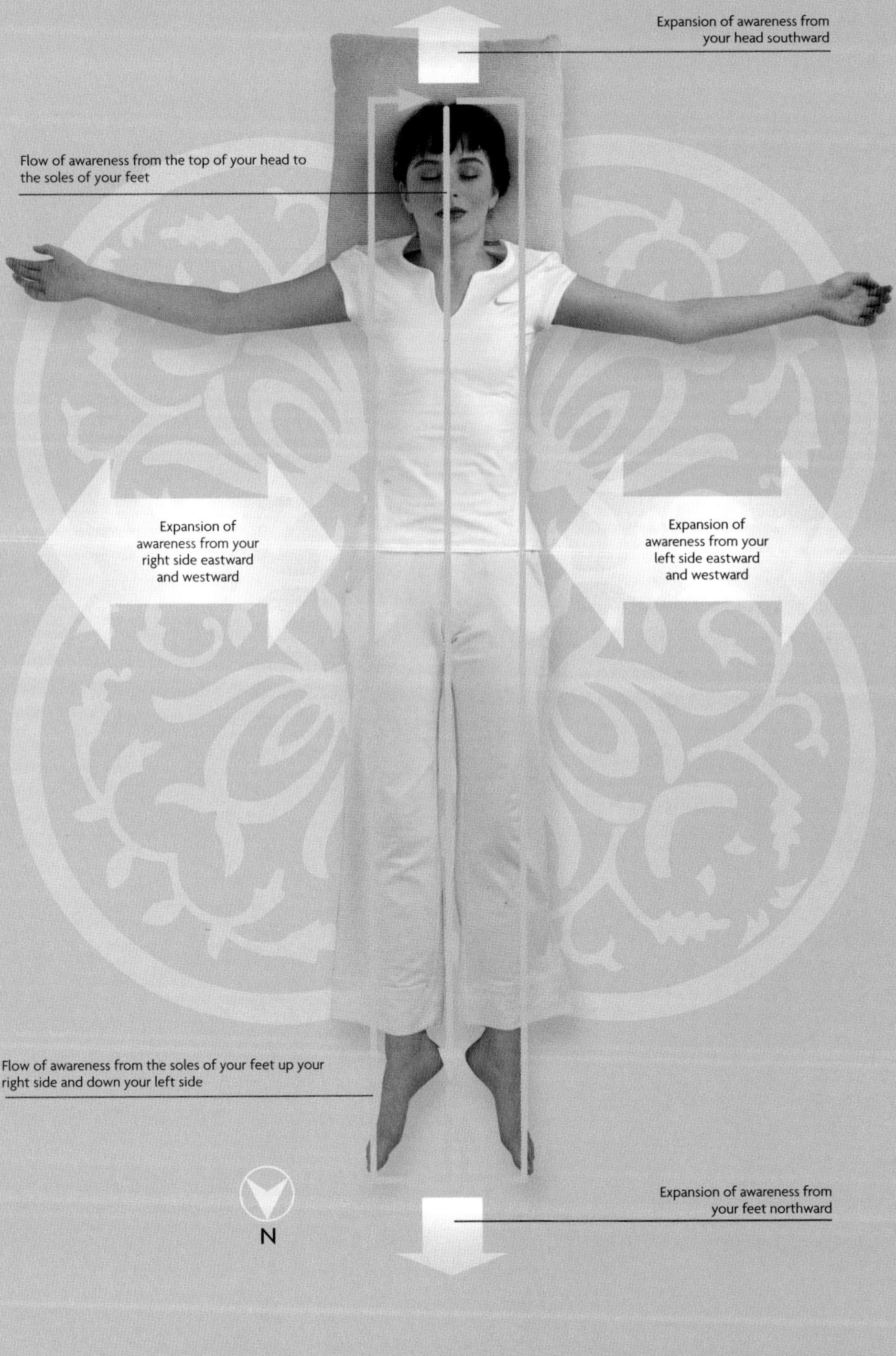

LEVEL: GREEN

Equalizing Male and Female Energy

In yoga, the male principle (sun energy) – known as Shiva – symbolizes consciousness and resides in the right side of the body, whereas the female principle (moon energy) – known as Shakti – is the activating power and resides in the left side of the body. Whenever you perform an action on one side of your body, such as breathing through one nostril or focusing your attention on one side or looking through one eye, it means you are focusing on and enhancing your mental awareness of either your male or your female energy. Then, when you change to the other side, you are consciously trying to stimulate the opposite energy, balancing the male and female energies within your body.

As an alternative to using an object (such as your thumb) as the focal point of this exercise, you can gaze at the tip of your nose, provided this does not strain your eye muscles. If you feel any strain or stinging during this exercise, close both eyes for a few minutes until they feel rejuvenated.

1 **Sit comfortably on the floor or on a chair. Place an object at eye level, preferably at a distance of 24 fingers. Close one eye and gaze at the object, making sure you do not strain your eye muscles.**

2 **Look until your eye gets tired but not strained. Let it close by itself when it is ready.**

3 **Open your other eye (keeping your first eye closed) and repeat the same gazing practice.**

4 Close both eyes. Go deep into your awareness and if any thoughts or feelings arise, simply observe them. To develop concentration and focus, keep doing this exercise for as long as you feel comfortable. Alternatively, you can move on to the next exercise: Shining the Light of Awareness.

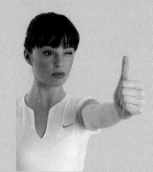

LEVEL: BLUE

Shining the Light of Awareness

Your brain tends to compartmentalize your feelings and emotions, likes and dislikes. Your subconscious is like a big house with different rooms, some of which have closed doors that you are hesitant to open. This meditation enables you to explore with absolute awareness every thought, every idea and every concept that is hiding behind a closed door or has been locked in a compartment by your subconscious mind. It is especially helpful if you think that negative feelings associated with past events are trapped inside you, enabling you to bring light and love to such emotions so you can look at them and accept them, realize that they can't hurt you, and ultimately allow them to leave.

1 Sit comfortably on the floor or on a chair. Close your eyes and start to explore the rooms in your mind. Perhaps you feel scared because you don't know what you will find when you open the doors. Observe each thought, feeling and emotion that enters your head and bring a sense of self-acceptance to your awareness. These things are a part of you, they are within your mind and your body. If you fight with them, you are fighting with yourself and this will deplete your energy.

2 Bring the light of your awareness to these thoughts, feelings and emotions so that they no longer remain hidden away – if you keep the doors open, they can leave when they are ready.

LEVEL: YELLOW

Meditation with the Eyes

It is often said that the eyes are the doorway to the soul as they take in so much information. The brain evaluates this data and sends messages to the rest of the body. When our perception changes inside, what we view outside often changes as well – although the same circumstances are present in our life, we see through 'new eyes' because our perception has shifted.

When you meditate with your eyes, you are sitting and watching at the crossover point between the outside world and your own inner world. First, you discover the duality that exists and then, once you have melted into accepting this, you realize that the source of everything is within you. And so the duality is unified.

The third eye is the seat of the ego and the self, and the place where all the chakras are connected. It is also one of the main sites from which samskaras are released. Your root chakra, your belly button and your third eye represent the three main points of your existence: your physical groundedness in your body; your source of life through your belly button; and the point of unification at the third eye. In this exercise you engage your root chakra, your belly button and your third eye at the same time, and so bring the different aspects of yourself together. This exercise will bring you physical and mental composure and a sense of confidence.

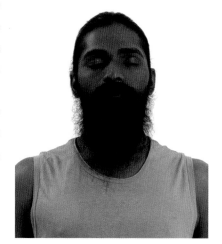

It is important to complete the final step of this exercise as this brings the energy you have created in your third eye back down through your body, creating equilibrium.

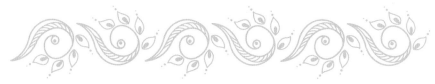

1 Sit comfortably on the floor or on a chair. Close your eyes and keep your eyes and face muscles relaxed. Notice your breath as it moves gently in and out of your nostrils. Make your inhalation the same length as your exhalation.

2 Bring your awareness to your eyes and look into the insides of your eyelids, gently and without straining. Try to keep your eyes from moving too much and 'looking around' inside – they should be as still as possible. You may experience colours or lighter or darker shades, or no colour at all – only the stillness. Whatever you experience, just observe it and accept it. There is no right or wrong thing to experience.

3 Now bring your awareness to placing your eyes as deeply as possible in their eye sockets and looking into the rest of your head – it's as if your eyeballs were turned inward. Without straining your eyes allow them to have a good look around inside your mind.

4 Remain with this practice for around 15 minutes.

5 Now take your gentle awareness to your third eye, without strain or effort – just the intention of your awareness. Next, take all your energy to your third eye and leave it there. You may experience different sensations such as light changes. Stay with your breath and remain at this point for approximately 10 minutes.

6 Now bring your awareness to your belly button, your root chakra and your anus, and engage all three points in combination with awareness/attention at your third eye. Remain here for around 5 minutes.

7 When you have completed the meditation, rub your palms together to generate heat and place them over your eyes. Gently open your eyes in your palms and smooth the energy over your face and your head. Massage your ears, smooth your aura down your chest to your stomach, down your back to your hips, over your hips to your thighs and to your calves and feet. Finally, massage your feet for a few moments.

LEVEL: GREEN

Stitching Together Left and Right

This practice (available as a download from www.yogiashokananda.com) can create an experience of kundalini or metatron and will help enormously if you feel that your body is unbalanced or that your energy is blocked when you try to meditate. It brings equal awareness of the left and right sides of your body and helps you to rejuvenate the energies of both sides of your body and hence both sides of your brain: female and male, moon and sun, ida and pingala, cold and heat, negative and positive. Think of the spine as a pillar in the centre of your body, connecting the two parts of your existence: your spirituality (pursa) and your physical self (prakriti). When universal and individual consciousness connect with each other through the spine, the state of pure consciousness is reached.

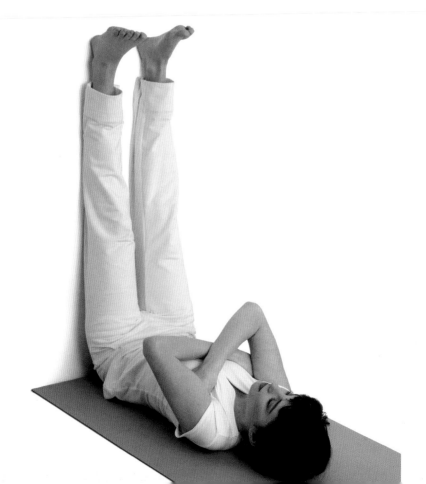

1 Lie down (preferably without a pillow), covering your body with a light blanket if necessary. Alternatively, raise your legs up against a wall with your tailbone also resting against the wall. Close your eyes.

2 Bring your whole awareness to the right side of your body – muscles, bones, circulation and brain. Feel that you have divided yourself in half. Connect to your organs, muscles and bones by looking and feeling, almost as if your mind is touching them, talking to them, relaxing them. Start by seeing and feeling the sensation of your right big toe ... travel slowly, slowly, to your heel and ankle ... feel the space ... travel up your calf to your knee, thigh and groin, the right side of your belly button, your sternum and lung, the right side of your heart, stomach, liver, bladder and back, your right shoulder and arm, the right side of your chest, throat, face and chin, your right ear, the right side of the back of your head, your eye and eyebrow, the right side of your teeth and lips, your right sinus, the right side of your forehead and brain, and finally your right nostril.

3 Practise inhaling and exhaling only through the right side of your body, as if only your right side exists. You are only conscious and aware of the male energy or the sun energy, the heat. As you inhale though your right nostril, feel that you are breathing only on the right side: through the right side of your forehead, the right side of your brain, your right neck, along the right side of your spine, the right side of your back, your right buttock, right kidney, right hip, right thigh, the right side of your rectum, your right knee, right calf and shin, and through your right ankle to your right foot. One inhalation is from nostril to toe.

4 Exhale through the right side of your body with the same awareness, from toe to nostril, until the last of your breath has been expelled. Your mind is travelling from your right foot through each part of the right side of your body. Continue breathing in this way until you are oblivious to the left side of your body but you are completely aware of your right side.

5 Now shift your awareness to your left side. See and feel the sensation of your left big toe ... travel slowly, slowly, to your heel and ankle ... feel the space ... travel up your calf to your knee, thigh and groin, the left side of your belly button, your sternum and lung, the left side of your heart, stomach, liver, bladder and back,

your left shoulder and arm, the left side of your chest, throat, face and chin, your left ear, the left side of the back of your head, your eye and eyebrow, the left side of your teeth and lips, your left sinus, the left side of your forehead and brain, and finally your left nostril.

6 Practise inhaling and exhaling only through the left side of your body, as if only your left side exists. You are only conscious and aware of the female energy or the moon energy, the coolness. As you inhale through your left nostril, feel that you are breathing only on the left side: through the left side of your forehead, the left side of your brain, your left neck, along the left side of your spine, the left side of your back, your left buttock, left kidney, left hip, left thigh, the left side of your rectum, your left knee, left calf and shin, and through your left ankle to your left foot. One inhalation is from nostril to toe.

7 Exhale through the left side of your body with the same awareness, from toe to nostril, until the last of your breath has been expelled. Your mind is travelling from your left foot through each part of the left side of your body. Continue practising until you become totally aware and rejuvenated in the left side of your body but have become oblivious to your right side.

8 Feel that your spine is the only thing that keeps your body together. All the nerves that come from your spine are connected to your organs. They are like stitches, holding your right and left sides together – sun and moon, yin and yang, male and female. Breathe along your spine from your tailbone up into the middle of your head and back down again. You are bringing equal awareness from the bottom to the top and from the top to the bottom of your spine. Each complete breath is giving energy to the nerves so they can bring right and left together and make you feel complete, and recharging the kundalini in your spine which carries a message from the lower to higher chakras, and from the higher to lower.

9 Stay with the experience of your breath and your spine until you feel the equilibrium of both energies in your mental, physical and energetic body.

10 When you are ready gently return to a comfortable sitting position. Feel the sense of freedom, light and openness in your spine – now free from blockages, it has been rebirthed and energized.

LEVEL: GREEN

Rising Sap

This profound meditation connects the opposing forces of the earth element of your body with the ether element (space) around you. It removes energy blockages and rejuvenates your mind and muscles by lifting the vibration of your body with the support of Mother Earth. When you do this exercise, it feels as if you are opening the channels in your body for the Divine Mother to recharge your body and bestow a sense of gravity on your life. If you are experiencing stress, lack of focus and an inability to make decisions, try this exercise as it is good for reducing the excessive vata (air element) that causes these symptoms. It is also an effective antidote for insomnia and depression, enabling you to connect with yourself and ground yourself in your environment.

During this practice (available as a download from www.yogiashokananda.com) you may feel a very heavy or tingling sensation in your whole body or a feeling that thousands of ants are running all over your skin. This is caused by the release of stress, the rejuvenation of your blood cells and the connection of your mind to your body. Sometimes people experience an almost orgasmic feeling as the Divine enters their body and unity occurs between two opposing forces: male and female, matter and spirit.

1   Sit on a chair or sofa with the soles of your bare feet flat and connected with the floor. If the floor is cold, you can place a cushion or pillow underneath your feet. Keep your palms relaxed in your lap and facing up, with your fingers naturally curled. Close your eyes softly.

2   Become aware of any space between your feet and the floor as well as the areas of contact. Where your feet are touching the floor, you feel that roots are growing into the ground, going deep into Mother Earth. Let your mind expand also to the centre of the earth. Like a tree you feel rooted. Your feet are heavy and grounded by the roots that are anchoring you to the Divine Mother and her nourishing, nurturing energy.

3   You are connected with an infinite and constant flow of energy. Once you have made this connection from deep within Mother Earth, a white, very light, milky cloud of energy starts enveloping the roots. As it reaches your feet you can feel it entering your body.

4   The energy keeps flowing into your feet from Mother Earth. The level rises up to your ankles, your calves and into your kneecaps and all around your knees. Now it is coursing through your whole body, continuing past your thighs into your hip cups, your groin, your rectum and urinary muscles, your tailbone, your lower back and your abdomen. Both legs are brimming with it.

5   The level rises up into your tummy – just relax your tummy and let it hold the energy like a pot. All your internal organs are filled and floating with this energy inside and outside of them. Let yourself go with the flow … the energy never ceases … it just keeps coming up through your feet into your legs, through your tummy, your back and up to your shoulders. From your shoulders it descends and fills your heart and chest and rolls down into your arms, to your palms, to the tip of your fingertips and into your palms.

6   You feel the energy shooting out from your fingertips. You feel balls of swirling energy in both palms.

7   Energy is still streaming continuously into your body from Mother Earth … milky white, very light nourishing energy … your feet, legs, belly, back and shoulders

are completely full. Now the level reaches your throat, your neck, your chin, your tongue, your teeth. It flows over your cheekbones, your ears and your eyes. Your eyelids are so relaxed and heavy, your eye muscles, sockets and nerves have no tension whatsoever. Your eyes can hardly open.

8 Now the level has reached your third eye, and you feel almost saturated by the milky white, cloudy energy from Mother Earth as it fills the top of your head. But then it pushes out from the top of your head like a fountain, as if bathing your body on its journey back to Mother Earth.

9 You are totally covered with this loving, tender, nourishing, healing energy from Mother Earth. It bathes your body inside and out, clearing all blockages and obstacles, easing strained muscles, regenerating and relaxing them. You feel that you are totally connected to Mother Earth. She is filling and regenerating your body and your mind with her energy.

10 You experience a sense of openness at the top of your head. Now the energy from the ether enters your body like a golden lightning bolt and unites with the earth's energy so you are recharged. You are fully aware and alert and are connected to both dimensions of your existence: higher and lower, heaven and earth. You feel that male and female, nature and spirit have united in your body. You feel complete and whole and totally loved and nourished.

11 In your own time slowly move your fingers and toes and place both palms on your heart chakra to acknowledge your existence with grace and gratitude – you experience a sense of openness and love, compassion for yourself and others, and a sense of letting go and release. You feel complete and whole, and filled with joy.

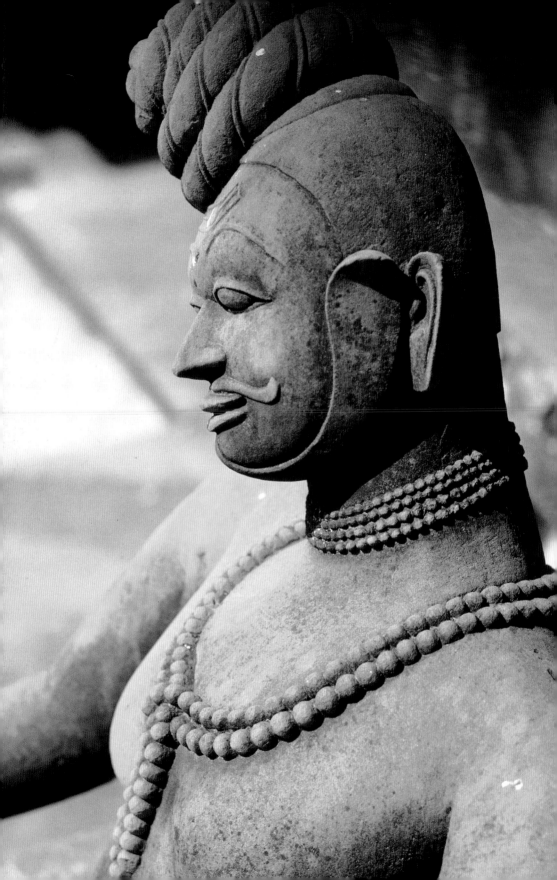

CHAPTER 6

Total Relaxation

This chapter summarizes what you have learned about the meaning of total relaxation and contains three meditations to help you complete your spiritual journey to your centre, to connect with universal energy. The Science of Relaxation™ meditation in particular is a powerful and transformational exercise that brings energy into the body on the breath and transports it to every part, releasing samskaras and healing the body and mind on every level.

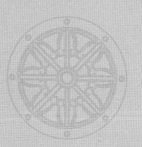

'Silence is a beautiful language. If more people spoke it,
the world would be a better place.'

YOGI ASHOKANANDA

Connecting to Our Infinite Source

Total relaxation is only possible when you completely surrender and are in your centre, your higher nature. Nothing can move you, nothing can knock you off-balance. But if you are living a life that is untrue to yourself (perhaps you have assumed a false personality or borrowed ideas), you will be haunted by insecurities and fears about what you may lose, no matter how loved and relaxed you think you are.

To be totally relaxed you have to bring all your five senses under your supervision – not under the supervision of society, not under the supervision of the intellect, but under the supervision of intelligence. Intelligence is not the same as intellect. The latter is specific to the mind and the senses, and can change. Intelligence, however, is the subject of the spirit or the soul and can never be changed but will always grow. By higher nature, soul or spirit, I mean an infinite source of intelligence or God. As we are part of this intelligence in the form of our body, senses, subtle body and spirit, all of these parts must be engaged in true relaxation.

If we put our intelligence into something, that something is filled with our intelligence. If we put our intelligence into something else, that too is filled. But it is all the same intelligence – there is only one. In the same way that a pot contains space, so a house contains space, and the sky contains space, and this space is all the same. And so all intelligence is identical and connected. In order to achieve total relaxation we must connect with this single, eternal, universal intelligence, which has no individual identity.

In a state of deep meditation, your mind loses sight of the external world. There is nothing but pure, infinite consciousness. Pure consciousness is the witness, and all that the witness sees is consciousness because that is all that exists. Once you reach that state, you will never feel fear because you will be connected with the true nature of yourself.

The Frog

The frog is like a human.
He constantly sticks his tongue out to eat flies,
Leaving his comfort zone,
Leaving his home to find satisfaction.
Before he knows it, he gets eaten by a snake.
So it is for us. We leave our eternal source,
Constantly wandering and searching like a frog,
We forget our awareness and we lose ourselves so much
That we get fascinated like a frog.
Before we know it, time eats us.
It is the nature of totality or a cycle.
If we are out of our centre,
If we are not at home,
We are all travellers, like tourists.
We come into the body and onto the earth as tourists.
Despite our father and our inner nature being so rich,
We seek pleasure and riches in foreign lands through our senses.
Our father in our nature kindly awaits to give us total richness
But our greed is never satisfied.
As tourists with limited permission to stay and explore
We put so much investment in foreign lands
Despite our father and our inner nature being so rich
The richness waits before us
When we feel pain and disappointment or the loss of investment in foreign lands
through the senses,
We feel hurt, we feel pain, we feel sorrow.
Despite our father and our inner nature being so rich.
Our minds have created so much confusion, our senses don't know what to follow.
Return to your home, which waits for you within your heart,
To the fullness of joy with the richness of fulfilment.
Return home to your inner nature
To rest at ease
With love and peace.

YOGI ASHOKANANDA

Finding Equilibrium

The only way to align and be balanced in your centre is by using your breath, engaging your body, surrendering and acknowledging and accepting the nature of duality. The practices I have described throughout this book distribute the life force, prana, throughout your body to balance your body and your mind. This chapter's meditations will help you to use your breath to move energy and blood flow into different organs, in order to bring about total equilibrium as well as releasing those soul memories and experiences (samskaras) that may be draining your energy.

As we have seen, samskaras are the remaining impressions left on your soul by experiences that form your personality. They are your unused emotions (your karma), which remain in your subconscious and have a profound influence on your physical and emotional state. Samskaras hold onto your energy, making you feel lethargic, stressed and anxious. They can even develop into chronic conditions and dis-ease. Remember: whatever emotion appears on a physical level will have appeared on an energetic level first.

You do not have to try to rid yourself of negativity – instead, you are shifting your perception and changing your physical body along with the memories it contains. In this way, even if the memory of something you once found traumatic may still be there, your reaction to it has been transformed.

Peace, bliss, freedom, joy, silence, happiness and whatever else you enjoy are all part of you and within you. You just need to make these things available to yourself. Being miserable takes up a lot of room in your mind, but you do not need to have a lot going on there in order to be happy!

THE RELEASE OF SAMSKARAS

There are two types of samskaras or stored memories, those deriving from the experiences of your past lives and those deriving from your present life – from the information fed to you by your senses. These are stored all over the body but they are released from two different centres, which must be activated before release can take place. These centres are the belly button, which releases samskaras from previous lives, and the third eye, which releases samskaras from this life and also acknowledges samskaras from previous lives. If you awaken your third eye and align it with your belly button, you will be able to release the samskaras from previous lives as well as those deriving from this life (see page 115).

The third eye is the point at which samskaras connect to the outside world to create a karma. Your perception and knowledge of, and connection to, the outer world occurs through your senses at the third eye. This means that if your third eye is not aligned with your intelligence, it is in the dark – in other words, it accumulates samskaras, makes judgments and takes decisions without awareness.

These samskaras are stored in every cell of your body and affect the functionality of all your organs, so any release of samskaras can be felt all over your body and in the mind as well. When a samskara is brought to a peak to be released, it explodes like a volcano and this explosion is usually accompanied by an emotional and/or physical reaction, such as crying, or a mental realization. After the eruption there is silence and the body and mind are able to truly relax and connect with each other.

Often if people cannot sleep, or suffer from depression, stress or other symptoms of unrest in body and mind, it is because samkaras have accumulated and they do not know how to release them. Every day we wash our bodies on the outside, but we do not think about cleaning ourselves emotionally or energetically. All the exercises in this chapter will encourage the release of samskaras.

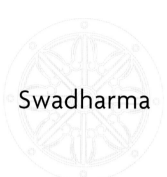

Swadharma

Swadharma means acting in accordance with your nature. To evolve, you need a personal revolution but this must be more than adopting the thoughts, ideas or actions of other people. Your inner revolution may contain the seeds of other people's ideas, but knowing your own purpose (your dharma) and being true to yourself are what really count. Even if you believe you have found your dharma by following somebody else's beliefs, your sense of purpose and contentment will not last for long. Awakening gives you the possibility to know yourself and your swadharma.

The only way to truly discover your dharma, to access your inner self and find total relaxation, peace and happiness is by practising meditation. You have already planted the seeds for that internal revolution by using the breathing techniques and various practices in this book.

The following three exercises will support you in discovering your true nature. Samskaras block your access to your true nature, but when they are released you are able to see yourself fully; in front of a metaphorical mirror, you stand absolutely naked and can see yourself as you are. You find the centre of yourself. When you are in your centre, you are unshakable, strong and gentle at the same time, and you are totally comfortable with your own uniqueness, which does not fit into any particular category or into anyone else's perception of you. You lose your self-consciousness but gain complete self-awareness.

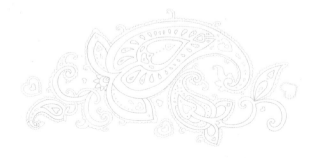

Atma Meditation

The Atma meditation is a meditation of the self, soul or spirit, which allows you to discover the infinite that exists within you – your inner power. It draws the power of the universe into you, aligning your individual self with universal energy and truth so you may come to realize your own reality. In so doing, your reality alters, as does your perception of your life. This means that real and important changes can now take place. Not only will you experience greater self-awareness, you will feel a greater connection to other people and to a higher source. Each and every one of us is entitled to feel inner peace, love, joy, fulfilment, happiness, freedom and success. This meditation allows you to access the power within you from which these experiences can develop and become a natural part of your life and who you are.

During this meditation focus your attention on the centre of your head. The centre of your brain is like the centre of the universe and because you want to access this place of infinity, you must keep your attention inside your mind, not outside your body. While you are meditating on the centre of your mind, feel the energy from the universe coming into this place and allow the universe to download its wisdom and infinite space into your head, your mind and your experience.

1 Sit comfortably on the floor or on a chair. Find the comfort of your own breath, your body and your mind. Bring your awareness to your whole physical body from your head to your fingertips and toes. Gently draw a little picture of your body in your mind and notice how you feel as you look at yourself.

2 Observe the serenity of your posture and let your mind experience the stillness. Don't try to create it, just sense the calm, the feelings of being still, of being open, of being free in your own self. You are meditating on your whole body rather than on the different parts. Your physical existence is inside your body, you are whatever you are, and right now you are looking at the dimension where you exist.

3 There is no pressure on your eyes to be closed. They are very gently shut because you are inside your whole body. Try to see yourself from six dimensions: top, bottom, front, back, left side and right side. There is nothing around you. You are alone with yourself.

4 You are at the centre of the wheel of life, of time. Let the light of universal energy rush toward you. Your brain is the centre of the universe and you are the vacuum drawing the whole universe into your body. Allow the universe to download its wisdom and infinite space into your mind. Continue to experience your own presence from all directions. Feel the energy of your awareness and sense the space. Stay with the feeling that you are the centre of everything, that everything is rushing into you and that everything ends inside you.

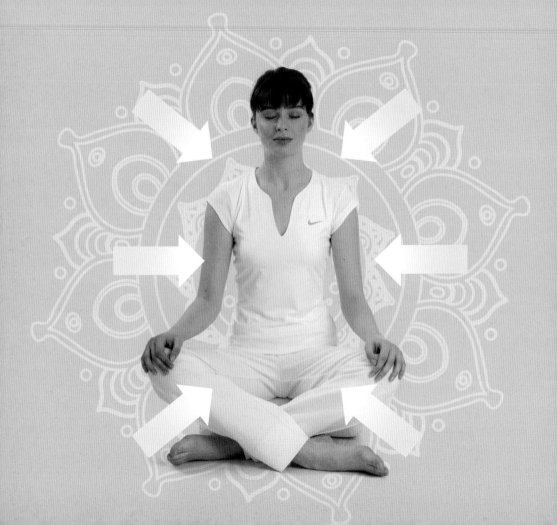

5 As thoughts and feelings arise, they rush into your body where they become diluted and disappear. Do not try to resist them as that only creates a divide where you are not with yourself. There is total acceptance. Whatever is coming, you are with your inner self. Absorb the light, the energy and the feelings rushing into you. You are the open space of the universe.

6 Gently place your hands over your heart and feel the warmth, the self-awareness, the love and compassion for yourself and for others. Experience feelings of grace and gratitude for your existence, and the sense of silence and clarity.

7 Smooth your aura down to your root chakra, and over your thighs to your feet. Rub your back, and then your arms from your shoulders to your fingertips.

8 Rub your hands together, place them in front of your face and let your eyes open gently in your palms. Place your hands on either side of your head and smooth the energy of your brain. Finish by gently stroking the back of your ears.

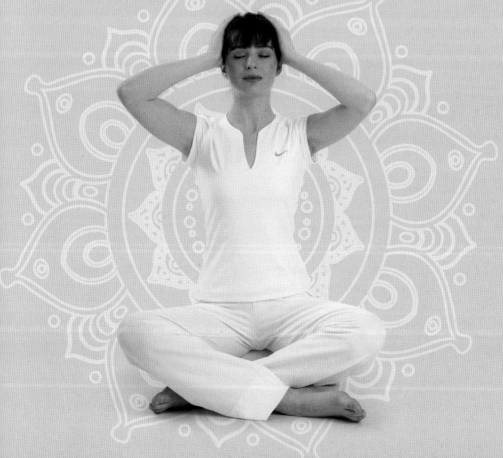

LEVEL: BLUE

Science of Relaxation™

This meditation has been described as a way of cleansing yourself from the inside out. We pay a lot of attention to caring for our bodies on the outside, but we must also look after the inner self and transform the energies that are not serving us well. When my teacher Gurudev Dilipji passed away in 2009, his wish was for the Science of Relaxation™ meditation to be brought to as many people as possible, so that they too could experience its transformational qualities. What makes this meditation so powerful is that it works on integrating all levels of your self – your material personality as well as your higher spiritual self. Its deep relaxation brings inner harmony and a revitalizing of mind and body. It replenishes feelings of optimism, openness and freedom and of being connected to yourself and others.

The Science of Relaxation™ breath connects your mind and your body. It surfaces, transforms and releases your emotions, while still retaining your energy. Letting go of past experiences and emotions frees you from your samskaras and the dis-eases within you. Negative and positive emotions are both part of your energy and your experience and they are both OK. This meditation allows you to explore your full personality and see all of yourself as you really are. Once your emotions have been set free, true relaxation can occur. It feels like the calm after the storm.

This meditation technique is one of the best antidotes for insomnia, depression, apathy and stress. It's generally good for mental health, the nervous system, blood pressure, the heart and digestion. Using breath awareness and control, it engages all the chakras and allows an even distribution of prana throughout the entire body, promoting an optimum state of health.

Practise this meditation as often as you can, though not more than twice a day. After doing it just once, many people report experiencing the sort of deep, restful sleep that they haven't enjoyed for years. Keep your eyes closed throughout to create maximum awareness of the energy in your body.

Swadharma

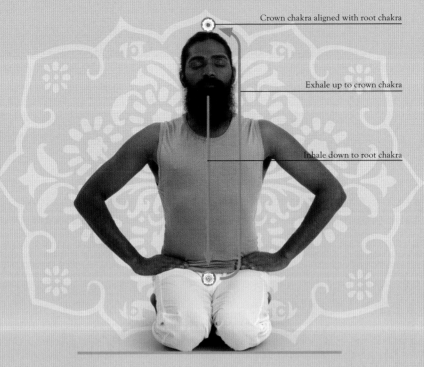

Crown chakra aligned with root chakra

Exhale up to crown chakra

Inhale down to root chakra

1 Sit on your heels, keeping your back straight. Relax your shoulders. Close your eyes and let your breath flow into your body. Bring your awareness into yourself as you inhale down to your root chakra and exhale upward into your head. The bottom and the top of your spine are aligned, and your root chakra is aligned with your crown chakra. Feel this connection.

2 Place your hands around your waist, with your forefingers pointing toward each other in front of your body and your thumbs pointing in the opposite direction. Your elbows are out to the sides.

3 Using ujayi breathing and keeping the tip of your tongue on the roof of your mouth, allow your breath to pass through the opening at the back of your throat.

4 Start to inhale for the count of one, two, three, four; hold for the count of five, six, seven, eight; then exhale for the count of seven, six, five, four, three, two, one. Do not force the breath – just allow it to pass gently and evenly. Repeat this eight times.

5 Now remove your hands from the waist and rest them in a comfortable position. Inhale and exhale deeply. Take another deep breath in. Exhale deeply. Take another deep breath in. Again, exhale deeply. Keep your eyes gently closed.

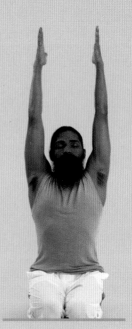

6 Now for the next phase: With a sharp inhalation, for 'one' throw your hands up, arms straight, palms facing each other and fingertips engaged and active. This allows your upper lungs to open and feeds your respiratory system with fresh oxygen. Imagine you are trying to lift your diaphragm and your back upward through the side of your ribcage.

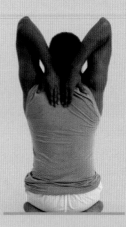

7 Exhale and on 'two' bring your hands back over your shoulders, elbows still bent, palms facing the back of your neck and fingers between your shoulder blades.

8 Now repeat this movement for the next 24 rounds of breath. After 24 rounds continue even faster if you can, synchronizing your breath with movement for another ten rounds of breath.

9 Inhale deeply and slowly, raising your arms up for the count of two, exhaling for the count of two. Repeat 24 times.

10 Release your arms down. Inhale deeply and exhale deeply. As you exhale, experience the openness, the vitality, the energy in your body, the sense of letting go, the sense of self-awareness, the feelings, the emotions, the sensations that arise in your head and your body.

11 Inhale into openness and vitality and inner space. Try to connect with your body and how you feel.

12 When you have completed the meditation, take 5 minutes (lie down if you can) to enjoying your inner space and openness, focusing equal awareness on your whole body and making sure that your whole body breathes to one heartbeat.

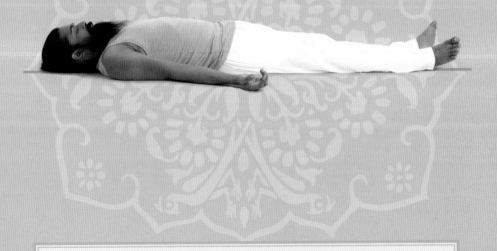

I sent my mind to get me a message
With my senses.
How did I know that my mind wouldn't disappear,
Taking my senses and getting lost in them?
I lost my senses, I lost my mind.
I don't know how to align.

YOGI ASHOKANANDA

LEVEL: ORANGE

Total Connection

This final practice can be done any time but is particularly effective after the Science of Relaxation™ meditation, as it connects your third eye (the seat of your ego) to your belly button (the root of your existence). You can now experience total relaxation, resting in a state of total you. Through this exercise you can shake off any false identity that you have assumed and feel completely confident in yourself.

1   Lie down comfortably and close your eyes. Inhale gently into your third eye. As the inhalation continues, gently direct your breath down to your belly button so the end of your inhalation ends there.

2   As you exhale, in your mind observe your breath as it travels up from your belly button and ends at your third eye.

3   Continue with this cycle for 10 minutes, keeping your eye muscles soft and relaxed, and your inhalation and exhalation natural and spontaneous.

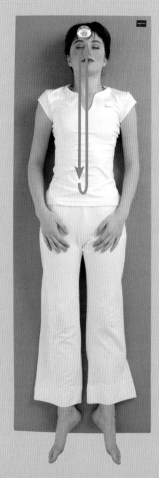

Some Personal Experiences
of the Practices

To understand how my approach to relaxation through yoga and meditation can help you physically, emotionally and spiritually, I am giving some space here to my students' own experiences of learning the practices described in this book. I hope you find their words inspiring.

'Soon after giving birth to my son, my mother became terminally ill and I unexpectedly faced motherhood as a single parent. Although I seemed on the outside to be coping, I remained in a state of grief and shock for almost four years, at which point I met Yogi again and began practising his techniques. From these, particularly the Science of Relaxation meditation and the exercise for breathing into the medulla, I learned to find a centre in myself again. I learned that patience and acceptance were key in moving on. I also learned to remain grounded in my body regardless of physical discomfort or emotional pain, to see myself more clearly and to reconnect to my heart. I accepted that the crumbling away of my old existence was part of my life's plan. Doing these meditations doesn't mean that life suddenly becomes easy and pain-free, but that you develop the inner strength to deal with whatever comes your way.' – *Mary, writer, mother, producer and co-founder of the Yogi Ashokananda School*

'Until I met Yogi, I was a very anxious, nervous person. I constantly judged myself and was uncomfortable expressing myself to others. Yogi uses relaxation techniques that guide you deep into the core of your existence. Here you can experience your true nature. Once I became familiar with my attachments I became less interested in them. I am now able to experience my life much more openly, express myself and share and receive love and knowledge, without false judgment holding me back. A whole new world has opened up for me.' – *Michelle, yoga teacher*

'By doing Yogi's pranayama and asana exercises, I have gained focus mentally and now have better control over my "monkey mind". Indeed, as I made a stronger commitment to my practice I found myself gaining strength both physically and professionally.' – *Paula, professor of law*

'Seventeen years ago my beloved son Jack suffered severe brain injury at birth. Yogi's exercises have helped me to learn how to disengage from my fears and go within, to reach a place less disturbed by anxiety, where I can connect with "who I really am". I pass on Yogi's teachings where possible to Jack. He particularly enjoys the Rising Sap meditation and regularly requests it. It gives him more awareness of his physical body and also reduces his spasms. We also use the breath techniques in hospital or during other stressful moments to help Jack tolerate invasive and painful procedures.' – *Karita, special needs teacher and therapist*

'My seven-year relationship had just broken down and I was also experiencing menopausal symptoms. I decided to attend Yogi's training. Now I enjoy my life much more, I am better able to deal with my commitments and responsibilities and my relationships generally have improved.' – *Jackie, beauty therapist and yoga teacher*

'I was holding onto trauma from my past, despite my chanting practice. I asked Yogi to help me. His powerful meditation techniques have moved mountains inside. I don't have the same level of pain any more and I feel much more connected. He also has given me clear guidance for dealing with obstacles in my path with calmness and inner strength.' – *Nikki, singer and voice coach*

'An auto-immune disease had left me with inflammation of the spinal cord. This caused epileptic-style fits in my legs and I was unable to control my bladder. Emotionally, I was in turmoil. Yogi's Science of Relaxation meditation was a great help to me as it calmed my nervous system, released a lot of tension and reduced the number of fits I had. At the same time I was able to improve my muscle tone and build up strength. Over a period of time my lungs got stronger and my awareness increased.' – *Apollonia, secretary and mother*

'I came to India to study Odissi dance but I was suffering from a back injury. Yogi selected the right practices to heal the injury and improve my whole physical condition and my ability to cope with my pain.' – *Yuval, professional classical Indian dancer*

Further Reading and Resources

Mascaró, Juan (trans.), **The Bhagavad Gita,** Penguin: London, 1962; new edition 2003

Venkatesananda, Swami (ed.), **The Supreme Yoga: Vashista Yoga**, Motilal Banarsidass: New Delhi, 2003

www.yogiashokananda.com

Visit this site for more information about Yogi's meditation, breathing and relaxation practices, as well as the Yogi Ashokananda School (offering weekly classes, workshops, retreats, private classes and teacher training). You can access free downloads of chanting and guided meditations from here, and buy Yogi's instructional DVDs: *Power Yoga & Kriya Yoga* and A.M. *(Solar) & P.M. (Lunar) Yoga.*

www.ashoktree.com

The Ashok Tree Ashram in Tiruvannamalai, Tamil Nadu, India, offers yoga, meditation and Ayurveda courses, retreats and teacher training.

www.atcharity.org

The Ashok Tree Foundation, Yogi's (UK-resistered) charity, offers yoga and meditation for stress management, helping those who want to help themselves. Classes in London are provided for students with mental or physical difficulties and for those of limited financial means. In India, the Ashok Tree Foundation offers education, health and hygiene services to communities in extreme poverty, and also provides a retreat centre and teacher-training programmes.

Index

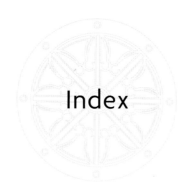

Index

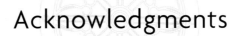

Acknowledgments

Author acknowledgments

I would like to acknowledge my teachers: Gurudev Dilipji, Masta Baba, Sri Lalji and Sri Krishna Ojha. I am grateful for the inspiration I have received from Swami Vivekananda, Dhirendra Brahmachari and Swami Vishnudevananda. And finally, my thanks to Mary Attwood for collecting and writing up my teachings for this book; she is a creative visionary!

Picture acknowledgments

The publisher would like to thank the following people, museums and photographic libraries for permission to reproduce their material. Every care has been taken to trace copyright holders. However, if we have omitted anyone we apologize and will, if informed, make corrections to any future edition.

Cover and page 1 Logo designed by Michael Parker; **page 2** Copyright © Images of India / Alamy; **page 7** Copyright © Jonathan Perugia; **page 11** Yogi Ashokananda; **page 16** Copyright © Neil McAllister / Alamy; **page 21** Roland and Sabrina Michaud; **page 25** Roland and Sabrina Michaud / akg-images; **page 27** Roland and Sabrina Michaud / akg-images; **page 43** Yogi Ashokananda; **page 46** Shutterstock; **page 49** Roland and Sabrina Michaud / akg-images; **page 63** Roland and Sabrina Michaud / akg-images; **page 68** Copyright © Peter M. Wilson / Alamy; **page 73** Copyright © Tim Gainey / Alamy; **page 81** Private Collection / Archives Charmet / Bridgeman Images; **page 98** Shutterstock; **page 101** akg-images / François Guénet; **pages 105–7** Shutterstock; **page 116** Copyright © dbimages / Alamy; **page 122** National Museum of India, New Delhi, India / Bridgeman Images; **page 138** Roland and Sabrina Michaud / akg-images